Lecture Notes: Respiratory Medicine

Lecture Notes
Respiratory Medicine

S.J. Bourke

MD, FRCPI, FRCP, FCCP, DCH
Consultant Physician
Royal Victoria Infirmary
Newcastle upon Tyne
Senior Lecturer in Medicine
University of Newcastle upon Tyne

Seventh Edition

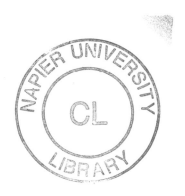

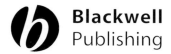
Blackwell
Publishing

First published 1975
Second edition 1980
Third edition 1985
Fourth edition 1991
Fifth edition 1998
Sixth edition 2003
Seventh edition 2007
1   2007

Library of Congress Cataloging-in-Publication Data

Bourke, S.J.
    Lecture notes. Respiratory medicine / S.J. Bourke. — 7th ed.
       p.; cm.
    Rev. ed. of: Lecture notes on respiratory medicine. 6th ed. 2003.
    Includes bibliographical references and index.
    ISBN-13: 978-1-4051-5344-7 (alk. paper)
    1. Respiratory organs—Diseases—Outlines, syllabi, etc.
  I. Bourke, S.J. Lecture notes on respiratory medicine. II. Title. III. Title: Respiratory medicine.
    [DNLM: 1. Respiratory Tract Diseases. WF 140 B8475L 2007]
    RC731.B69 2007
    616.2—dc22
2006032550

A catalogue record for this title is available from the British Library

Set in 8/12 Stone Serif by Charon Tec Ltd (A Macmillan Company), Chennai, India
www.charontec.com
Printed and bound in Singapore by Markono Print Media Pte Ltd

Commissioning Editor: Vicki Noyes
Editorial Assistant: Ellie Bonnet
Development Editor: Karen Moore
Production Controller: Debbie Wyer

For further information on Blackwell Publishing, visit our website:
http://www.blackwellpublishing.com

The publisher's policy is to use permanent paper from mills that operate a sustainable forestry policy, and which has been manufactured from pulp processed using acid-free and elementary chlorine-free practices. Furthermore, the publisher ensures that the text paper and cover board used have met acceptable environmental accreditation standards.

Contents

Preface

It is now more than 30 years since the first edition of *Lecture Notes on Respiratory Medicine* was written by my predecessor and colleague, Dr Alistair Brewis. It rapidly became a classic textbook which opened the eyes of generations of students to the special fascinations of the subject such that many were attracted into the specialty. Thus, students became teachers, and continued to learn by teaching. Subsequent editions show how respiratory medicine has developed over the years to become such a major specialty in hospitals and in the community, treating a wide range of diseases from cystic fibrosis to lung cancer, asthma to tuberculosis, sleep disorders to occupational lung diseases.

In the seventh edition the text has been revised and expanded to provide a concise up-to-date summary of respiratory medicine for undergraduate students and junior doctors preparing for postgraduate examinations. A particular feature of respiratory medicine in recent years has been the focusing of skills from a variety of disciplines in providing the best care for patients with respiratory diseases, and this book should be useful to colleagues such as physiotherapists, lung function technicians and respiratory nurse specialists. Some of Dr Alistair Brewis' original drawings have been retained. The emphasis of *Lecture Notes on Respiratory Medicine* has always been on information which is useful and relevant to everyday clinical medicine, and the seventh edition remains a patient-based book to be read before and after visits to the wards and clinics where clinical medicine is learnt and practised. As *Lecture Notes on Respiratory Medicine* develops over time, we remain grateful to our teachers and their teachers, and we pass on our evolving knowledge of respiratory medicine to our students and their students.

S.J. Bourke

Part 1

Structure and Function

Chapter 1

Anatomy and physiology of the lungs

Introduction

The essential function of the lungs is the **exchange of oxygen and carbon dioxide between the blood and the atmosphere**. This takes place by a process of molecular diffusion across the alveolar capillary membrane which has a surface area of about $60\,m^2$. The anatomy and physiology of the respiratory system are designed in such a way as to bring air from the atmosphere and blood from the circulation into close contact across the alveolar capillary membrane. Contraction of the diaphragm and intercostal muscles results in expansion of the chest and a fall in intrathoracic pressure which draws atmospheric air containing 21% oxygen into the lungs. **Ventilation** of the alveoli depends upon the size of each breath (tidal volume), respiratory rate, resistance of the airways to airflow and compliance (distensibility) of the lungs. About a quarter of the air breathed in remains in the conducting airways and is not available for gas exchange: this is referred to as the anatomical deadspace. The lungs are **perfused** by almost all the cardiac output from the right ventricle. There is a complex and dynamic interplay between ventilation and perfusion in maintaining gas exchange in health, and derangement of these parameters is a key pathophysiological feature of respiratory disease. Ventilation of alveoli which are not perfused increases deadspace, and blood passing from the pulmonary artery to the left atrium without passing through ventilated alveoli does not contribute to gas exchange, thereby forming a physiological shunt.

Bronchial tree

The **trachea** has cartilaginous horseshoe-shaped 'rings' supporting its anterior and lateral walls. The posterior wall is flaccid and bulges forward during coughing. The trachea divides into the right and left main bronchi at the level of the sternal angle (angle of Louis). The **left main bronchus** is longer than the right and leaves the trachea at a more abrupt angle. The **right main bronchus** is more directly in line with the trachea so that inhaled material tends to enter the right lung more readily than the left. The main bronchi divide into **lobar bronchi** (upper, middle and lower on the right; upper and lower on the left) and then **segmental bronchi** as shown in Fig. 1.1. The position of the lungs in relation to external landmarks is shown in Fig. 1.2. **Bronchi** are airways with cartilage in their walls, and there are about 10 divisions of bronchi beyond the tracheal bifurcation. Smaller airways without cartilage in their walls are referred to as **bronchioles**. **Respiratory bronchioles** are peripheral bronchioles with alveoli in their walls. Bronchioles immediately proximal to alveoli are known as **terminal bronchioles**. In the bronchi, smooth muscle is arranged in a spiral fashion internal to the cartilaginous plates. The muscle coat

3

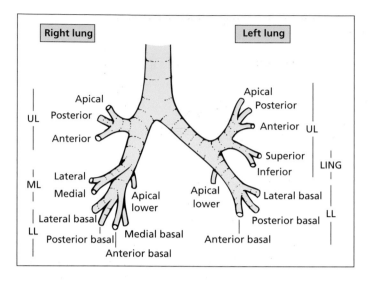

Right lung

Left lung

Apical
Posterior
UL
Anterior

Apical
Posterior
Anterior UL
Superior
Inferior LING

Lateral
ML
Medial

Apical
lower
Apical
lower
Lateral basal

Lateral basal
LL
Posterior basal

LL
Posterior basal Medial basal
Anterior basal

Anterior basal

Figure 1.1 Diagram of bronchopulmonary segments. LING, lingula; LL, lower lobe; ML, middle lobe; UL, upper lobe.

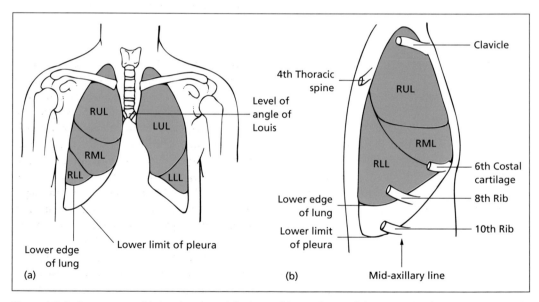

Clavicle

4th Thoracic spine

RUL

Level of angle of Louis

RUL

LUL

RML

RML

RLL

6th Costal cartilage

RLL

LLL

8th Rib

Lower edge of lung

Lower limit of pleura

10th Rib

Lower edge of lung

Lower limit of pleura

(a)

(b)

Mid-axillary line

Figure 1.2 Surface anatomy. (a) Anterior view of the lungs. (b) Lateral view of the right side of chest at resting end-expiratory position. LLL, left lower lobe; LUL, left upper lobe; RLL, right lower lobe; RML, right middle lobe; RUL, right upper lobe.

becomes more complete distally as the cartilaginous plates become more fragmentary. The epithelial lining is ciliated and includes goblet cells. The cilia beat with a whip-like action, and waves of contraction pass in an organised fashion from cell to cell so that material trapped in the sticky mucus layer above the cilia is moved upwards and out of the lung. This mucociliary escalator is an important part of the lung's defences. Larger bronchi also have acinar mucus-secreting glands in the submucosa which are hypertrophied in chronic bronchitis. **Alveoli** are about 0.1–0.2 mm in diameter and are lined

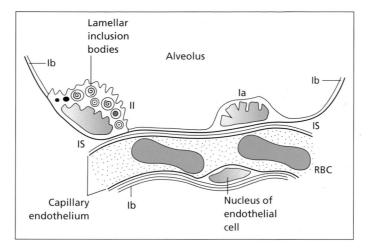

Figure 1.3 Structure of the alveolar wall as revealed by electron microscopy. Ia, type I pneumocyte; Ib, flattened extension of type I pneumocyte covering most of the internal surface of the alveolus; II, type II pneumocyte with lamellar inclusion bodies which are probably the site of surfactant formation; IS, interstitial space; RBC, red blood corpuscle. Pneumocytes and endothelial cells rest upon thin continuous basement membranes which are not shown.

by a thin layer of cells of which there are two types: type I pneumocytes have flattened processes which extend to cover most of the internal surface of the alveoli; type II pneumocytes are less numerous and contain lamellated structures which are concerned with the production of surfactant (Fig. 1.3). There is a potential space between the alveolar cells and the capillary basement membrane which is only apparent in disease states when it may contain fluid, fibrous tissue or a cellular infiltrate.

Alveolar ventilation

During **inspiration** the diaphragm descends, the lower ribs move upwards and outwards, and the upper ribs and sternum move upwards and forwards. The resultant expansion of the chest results in a negative intrathoracic pressure sucking air into the lungs. **Expiration**, by comparison, is a relatively passive procedure as the respiratory muscles gradually relax their force of contraction. About 8 L of air are drawn into the lungs each minute at rest but not all this air reaches the alveoli. About a quarter of the air breathed in remains in the airways from the trachea to the terminal bronchioles and is not available for gas exchange. This is referred to as

the **anatomical deadspace**. The distribution of air within the lungs is uneven because the resistance of the airways to airflow is not uniform and because the compliance of different parts of the lungs varies. The greater part of total **airway resistance** to airflow during inspiration in the normal individual occurs in the larger airways—trachea, main bronchi, larynx. Increased resistance occurring in disease generally originates in the more peripheral airways. During inspiration, pulmonary elastic recoil acts as a force opening the airways. During expiration, the outward traction on the walls of the airways diminishes so that there is an increasing tendency towards closure of the airways. **Compliance** is a physiological term expressing the distensibility of the lungs. The inherent elastic properties of the lungs cause them to retract from the chest wall producing a negative intrapleural pressure. Lung compliance is expressed as *the change in lung volume brought about by unit change in transpulmonary (intrapleural) pressure*. The retractive forces of the lung are balanced by the semi-rigid structure of the thoracic cage and the action of the respiratory muscles. The effect of gravity results in the weight of the lungs keeping the upper parts under a greater stretch than the more dependent zones. The upper parts are less compliant and less receptive to air entry during inspiration. Thus, the lower zones receive more ventilation than the upper zones. Local differences in compliance and airway resistance are present to a small degree even in normal lungs but occur to a much greater extent in diseased lungs.

Lung perfusion

The lungs receive a blood supply from both the pulmonary and systemic circulations. The **pulmonary artery** arises from the right ventricle and divides into left and right pulmonary arteries, which further divide into branches accompanying the bronchial tree. The pulmonary capillary network in the alveolar walls is very dense and provides a very large surface area for gas exchange. The pulmonary venules drain laterally to the periphery of lung lobules and then pass centrally in the interlobular and intersegmental septa, ultimately joining to form the four main pulmonary veins which empty into the left atrium. Several small **bronchial arteries** usually arise from the descending aorta and travel in the outer layers of the bronchi and bronchioles supplying the tissues of the airways down to the level of the respiratory bronchiole. Most of the blood drains into radicles of the pulmonary vein contributing a small amount of desaturated blood which accounts for part of the 'physiological shunt' observed in normal individuals. The bronchial arteries may undergo hypertrophy when there is chronic pulmonary inflammation, and major haemoptysis in diseases such as bronchiectasis or aspergilloma usually arises from the bronchial rather than the pulmonary arteries and may be treated by therapeutic bronchial artery embolisation. The pulmonary circulation normally offers a much lower resistance and operates at a lower perfusion pressure than the systemic circulation. At rest in the erect position, gravity exerts a major effect on the distribution of blood with perfusion being preferentially distributed to the lung bases. Hypoxia is a potent stimulus to pulmonary vasoconstriction and seems to exert a direct effect on arterial smooth muscle. This reflex acts as a form of autoregulation, diverting blood away from

underventilated areas of the lung. The pulmonary capillaries may also be compressed as they pass through the alveolar walls if alveolar pressure rises above capillary pressure.

Gas exchange and ventilation/perfusion (V/Q) relationships

During steady-state conditions the relationship between the amount of carbon dioxide produced by the body and the amount of oxygen absorbed depends upon the metabolic activity of the body and is referred to as the **respiratory quotient (RQ)**. The actual value varies from 0.7 during pure fat metabolism to 1.0 during pure carbohydrate metabolism. The RQ is usually about 0.8 but it is often assumed to be 1.0 to make calculations easier.

If carbon dioxide is being produced by the body at a constant rate the P_{CO_2} of alveolar air depends upon the amount of outside air that the carbon dioxide is mixed with in the alveoli, that is P_{CO_2} depends only upon alveolar ventilation and **arterial P_{CO_2} is a measure of alveolar ventilation**. If alveolar ventilation falls, P_{CO_2} rises. The level of alveolar P_{O_2} also varies with alveolar ventilation but measurement of arterial P_{O_2} is less reliable than measurement of P_{CO_2} as an index of alveolar ventilation because it is profoundly affected by regional changes in ventilation/perfusion ratios.

The possible combinations of P_{CO_2} and P_{O_2} are shown in Fig. 1.4. Moist atmospheric air at 37°C has a P_{O_2} of about 20 kPa (150 mmHg). In this model, oxygen could be exchanged with carbon dioxide in the alveoli to produce any combination of P_{O_2} and P_{CO_2} described by the oblique line which joins P_{O_2} 20 kPa (150 mmHg) and P_{CO_2} 20 kPa (150 mmHg). The position of the cross on this line represents the composition of a hypothetical sample of alveolar air. A fall in alveolar ventilation would result in an upward movement of this point along the line and conversely an increase in alveolar ventilation would result in a downward movement of the point. Point (a) represents the P_{CO_2} and P_{O_2} of arterial blood (it lies a little to the left of the RQ 0.8 line because of the small normal alveolar–arterial oxygen tension difference). Point (b)

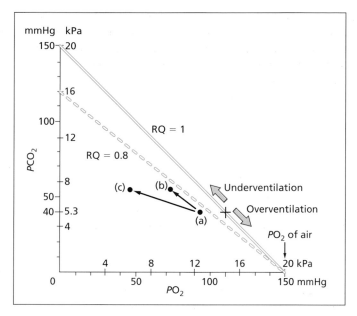

Figure 1.4 Oxygen–carbon dioxide diagram. The continuous and interrupted lines describe the possible combinations of P_{CO_2} and P_{O_2} in alveolar air when the RQ is 1 and 0.8, respectively. (a) A hypothetical sample of arterial blood. (b) Progressive underventilation. (c) Po2 lower than can be accounted for by underventilation alone.

represents the arterial gas tension after a period of underventilation. If the arterial P_{CO_2} and P_{O_2} were those represented by point (c) this would imply that the fall in P_{O_2} was more than could be accounted for on the grounds of reduced alveolar ventilation.

There is normally a small difference (<2.5 kPa or 20 mmHg) between alveolar and arterial oxygen tensions. This gradient may be roughly calculated using the simplified formula:

$$\text{Alveolar} - \text{arterial (A} - \text{a) gradient} = P_IO_2 - (P_O_2 + P_{CO_2})$$

(P_IO_2 is the partial pressure of fractional inspired oxygen which for atmospheric air at 37°C is 20 kPa).

The quantity of gas carried by blood when exposed to different partial pressures of the gas is described by the dissociation curve. The dissociation curves for oxygen and carbon dioxide are very different and are shown together on the same scale in Fig. 1.5. Over the range normally encountered the amount of carbon dioxide carried by the blood is roughly proportional to the P_{CO_2}. However, the quantity of oxygen carried is roughly proportional

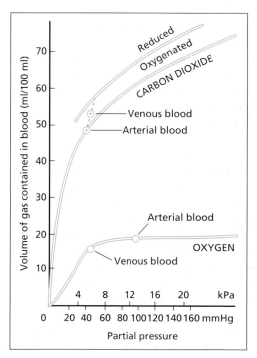

Figure 1.5 The blood oxygen and carbon dioxide dissociation curves drawn to the same scale.

to the P_{O_2} only over a very limited range of about 3–7 kPa (22–52 mmHg). Above 13.3 kPa (100 mmHg) the haemoglobin is fully saturated and hardly any additional oxygen is carried. The different shapes of the dissociation curves of oxygen and carbon dioxide explain why ventilation/perfusion mismatch has a greater effect on P_{O_2} than on P_{CO_2} levels.

Control of breathing

The **respiratory centre** in the brain stem consists of an ill-defined group of interconnected neurones, responsible for generating phasic motor discharges which ultimately pass via phrenic and intercostal nerves to the respiratory muscles. Some of the more important factors influencing the output of the respiratory centre are shown in Fig. 1.6. The P_{CO_2} of arterial blood is the most important factor in the regulation of ventilation. An **increase in P_{CO_2}**

stimulates sensitive areas on the surface of the brain stem directly provoking an increase in ventilation. An **increase in [H⁺]** (fall in pH) also stimulates ventilation. **Hypoxaemia** sensitises the respiratory centre to carbon dioxide probably via an effect on the carotid and aortic bodies. However, the effect of hypoxaemia is small above a P_{O_2} of about 8.8 kPa (60 mmHg). Input from **higher centres** is important, with alarm and excitement stimulating ventilation, and sleep and coma reducing the response to normal ventilatory stimuli. The **vagus nerve** carries afferent stimuli from the respiratory tract which may influence breathing. In animals, stretching of the lungs causes reflex inhibition of subsequent inspiration (Hering–Breuer inflation reflex) although the importance of this reflex is doubtful in humans. Stimulation of **J receptors**, situated deep in the lung parenchyma, increases ventilation. Excitation of stretch receptors in muscles, joints and chest wall may also enhance ventilation.

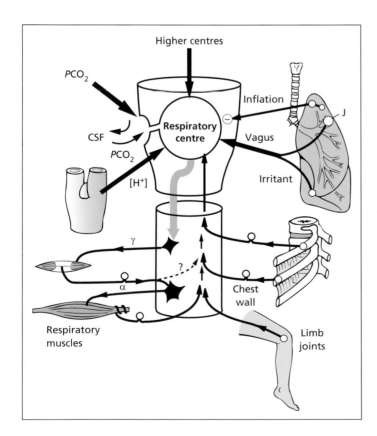

Figure 1.6 Control of ventilation: some of the more important factors involved (see text).

Keypoints

- The essential function of the lungs is the exchange of oxygen and carbon dioxide between the blood and the atmosphere.
- Ventilation is the process of drawing oxygen into the lungs, and it depends on the tidal volume, respiratory rate, resistance of the airways and the compliance of the lungs.
- Derangement in the matching of ventilation and perfusion in the lungs is an important factor causing hypoxia in lung disease.
- The respiratory centre in the brain stem is responsible for the control of breathing, and an increase in P_{CO_2} stimulates ventilation.

Further reading

Brewis RAL, White FE. Anatomy of the thorax. In: Gibson GJ, Geddes DM, Costabel U, Sterk PJ, Corrin B, eds. *Respiratory Medicine*. Edinburgh: Elsevier Science Ltd. 2003: 3–33.

Cotes JE. *Lung Function: Assessment and Application in Medicine*. Oxford: Blackwell Science, 1993.

Gibson GJ. *Clinical Tests of Respiratory Function*. Oxford: Chapman and Hall, 1996.

West JB. *Pulmonary Pathophysiology—The Essentials*. Baltimore, MD: Williams and Wilkins, 1987.

Part 2

History Taking, Examination and Investigations

Chapter 2

History taking and examination

History taking

History taking is of paramount importance in the assessment of a patient with respiratory disease. Difficult diagnostic problems are more often solved by a carefully taken history than by laboratory tests. It is during history taking that the doctor also gets to know the patient and the patient's fears and concerns. The relationship of trust thus established forms the basis of the therapeutic partnership. Start by asking the patient to describe the symptoms in his or her own words. Listening to the patient's account of the symptoms is an active process in which the doctor is seeking clues to underlying processes, judging which items require further exploration and noting the patient's attitude and anxieties. By carefully posed questions the skilled clinician directs the patient to focus on pertinent points, to clarify crucial details and to explore areas of possible importance. History-taking skills develop with experience and with a greater knowledge of respiratory disease.

It is important to appreciate the differences between **symptoms**, which are a patient's subjective description of a change in the body or its functions which may indicate disease, **signs**, which are abnormal features noted by the doctor on examination and **tests**, which are objective measurements undertaken at the bedside or in the diagnostic laboratories. Thus, for example, a patient might complain of pain on breathing, the doctor might elicit tenderness on pressing on the chest and an X-ray might show a fractured rib.

Symptoms (Table 2.1)

Dyspnoea

This is an unpleasant sensation of **being unable to breathe easily** (i.e. breathlessness). Analysis of this symptom requires an assessment of the speed of onset, progression, periodicity and precipitating and relieving factors. The severity of dyspnoea is graded according to the patient's exercise tolerance (e.g. dyspnoeic on climbing a flight of stairs; dyspnoeic at rest). Onset may be sudden as in the case of a pneumothorax, or gradual and progressive as in chronic obstructive pulmonary disease (COPD). An episodic dyspnoea pattern is characteristic of asthma with symptoms typically being precipitated by cold air or exercise. **Orthopnoea** is dyspnoea which occurs when lying flat and is

Table 2.1 Main respiratory symptoms.

- Dyspnoea
- Wheeze
- Cough
- Sputum
- Haemoptysis
- Chest pain

relieved by sitting upright. It is a characteristic feature of pulmonary oedema or diaphragm paralysis but is found also in many respiratory diseases. **Paroxysmal nocturnal dyspnoea** (PND) refers to the phenomenon of the patient waking up breathless at night. It is most commonly associated with pulmonary oedema but must be distinguished from the nocturnal wheeze and the sleep disturbance of asthma. It is important to note what words the patient uses to describe the symptoms: 'tightness in the chest' may indicate breathlessness or angina. Dyspnoea is not a symptom which is specific to respiratory disease and it may be associated with various cardiac diseases, anxiety, anaemia and metabolic states such as ketoacidosis.

Wheeze

This is a whistling or sighing noise which is characteristic of air passing through a narrow tube. The sound of wheeze can be mimicked by breathing out almost to residual volume and then giving a further sharp forced expiration. Wheeze is a characteristic feature of airways obstruction caused by asthma or COPD but can also occur in pulmonary oedema. In asthma, wheeze is characteristically worse on waking in the morning and may be precipitated by exercise or cold air. Wheeze which improves at weekends or on holidays away from work and deteriorates on return to the work environment is suggestive of occupational asthma. In asthma and COPD wheezing is more prominent in expiration. An inspiratory wheeze—**stridor**—is a feature of disease of the central airways (e.g. obstruction of the trachea by a carcinoma).

Cough and sputum

Cough is a forceful expiratory blast produced by contraction of the abdominal muscles with bracing by the intercostal muscles and sudden opening of the glottis. It is a protective reflex which removes secretions or inhaled solid material, and it is provoked by physical or chemical stimulation of irritant receptors in the larynx, trachea or bronchial tree. Cough may be dry or associated with sputum production. The duration and nature

of the cough should be assessed, and precipitating and relieving factors explored. It is important to examine any **sputum** produced, noting whether it is mucoid, purulent or bloodstained, for example. Cough occurring on exercise or disturbing sleep at night is a feature of asthma. A transient cough productive of purulent sputum is very common in respiratory tract infections. A weak ineffective cough which fails to clear secretions from the airways is a feature of bulbar palsy or expiratory muscle weakness, and predisposes the patient to aspiration pneumonia. Cough is often triggered by the accumulation of sputum in the respiratory tract. Chronic bronchitis is defined as cough productive of sputum on most days for at least 3 months of 2 consecutive years. Bronchiectasis is characterised by the production of copious amounts of purulent sputum. A chronic cough may also be caused by gastro-oesophageal reflux with aspiration, sinusitis with post-nasal drip and occasionally by drugs (e.g. captopril). Violent coughing can generate sufficient force to produce a '**cough fracture**' of a rib or to impede venous return and cerebral perfusion causing '**cough syncope**'. Patients with alveolar cell carcinoma sometimes produce very large volumes of watery sputum: **bronchorrhoea**. Patients with coalworker's pneumoconiosis will occasionally cough up black material: **melanoptysis**.

Haemoptysis

This is the **coughing up of blood**. It is a very important symptom which requires investigation. In particular, it may be the first clue to the presence of bronchial carcinoma, and early investigation may detect the tumour at a stage when curative surgery can be performed. All patients with haemoptysis should have a chest X-ray performed, and further investigations such as bronchoscopy, computed tomography (CT), sputum cytology and microbiology may be indicated depending on the circumstances. The most important causes of haemoptysis are bronchial carcinoma, lung infections (pneumonia, bronchiectasis, tuberculosis), chronic bronchitis, pulmonary infarction, pulmonary oedema and pulmonary vasculitis (Table 2.2). In some cases no cause is found and the origin of the blood

Table 2.2 Major causes of haemoptysis.

Tumours
- Bronchial carcinoma
- Laryngeal carcinoma

Infections
- Tuberculosis
- Pneumonia
- Bronchiectasis
- Infective bronchitis

Infarction
- Pulmonary embolism

Pulmonary oedema
- Left ventricular failure
- Mitral stenosis

Pulmonary vasculitis
- Goodpasture's syndrome
- Wegener's granulomatosis

may have been in the upper airway (e.g. nose (epistaxis), pharynx or gums).

Chest pain

Pain which is aggravated by inspiration or coughing is described as **pleuritic pain**, and the patient can often be seen to wince when breathing in, as the pain 'catches'. Irritation of the pleura may result from inflammation (pleurisy), infection (pneumonia), infarction of underlying lung (pulmonary embolism) or tumour (malignant pleural effusion). Chest wall pain resulting from injury to the intercostal muscles or fractured ribs, for example, is also aggravated by inspiration or coughing and is associated with tenderness at the point of injury.

In addition to these major respiratory symptoms it is important to consider other associated symptoms. For example, **anorexia** and **weight loss** are features of malignancy or chronic lung infections (e.g. lung abscess). **Pyrexia** and **sweating** are features of acute (e.g. pneumonia) and chronic infections (e.g. tuberculosis). **Lethargy**, malaise and confusion may be features of hypoxaemia. **Headaches**, particularly on awakening in the morning, may be a symptom of hypercapnia. **Oedema** may indicate cor pulmonale. **Snoring** and daytime **somnolence** may indicate obstructive sleep apnoea syndrome. **Hoarseness** of the voice may

indicate damage to the recurrent laryngeal nerve by a tumour.

Many respiratory diseases have their roots in previous **childhood lung disease** or in the **patient's environment** so that it is crucial to make specific enquiries concerning these points during history taking.

History

Past medical history

Did the patient suffer any major illness in childhood? Did the patient have frequent absences from school? Was the patient able to play games at school? Did any abnormalities declare themselves at a pre-employment medical examination or on chest X-ray? Has the patient ever been admitted to hospital with chest disease? A long history of childhood 'bronchitis' may in fact indicate asthma. Severe whooping cough or measles in childhood may cause bronchiectasis. Tuberculosis acquired early in life may re-activate many years later.

General medical history

Has the patient any systemic illness which may involve the lungs (e.g. rheumatoid arthritis)? Is the patient taking any medications which might affect the lungs (e.g. amiodarone), which can cause interstitial lung disease, or β-blockers (e.g. atenolol), which may provoke bronchospasm? What effect will the patient's lung disease have on other illnesses (e.g. fitness for surgery?).

Family history

Is there any history of lung disease in the family? An increased prevalence of lung disease in a family may result from 'shared genes', that is inherited traits such as cystic fibrosis, α_1-anti-trypsin deficiency, asthmatic tendency; or from 'shared environment' (e.g. tuberculosis).

Social history

Does the patient smoke, or has he or she ever smoked? Is the patient exposed to passive smoking

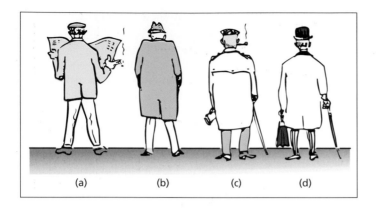

Figure 2.1 Which man has airways obstruction? (Answer at foot of p. 17.)

at home? It is important to obtain a clear account of total smoking exposure over the years so as to assess the patient's risk for diseases such as lung cancer or COPD. Does the patient keep any pets or participate in any sports (e.g. diving) or hobbies (e.g. pigeon racing) which may be important in assessing the lung disease?

Occupational history

What occupations has the patient had over the years, what tasks were performed and what materials used? Did symptoms show a direct relationship to the work environment as in the case of occupational asthma improving away from work and deteriorating on return to work? Has the patient been exposed to substances which may give rise to disease many years later as in the case of mesothelioma arising from exposure to asbestos 20–40 years previously?

Examination

Examination of the respiratory system is, of course, integrated into the general examination of the patient as a whole, but outlining the different stages in the assessment of the respiratory system is useful in focusing attention on the features of particular importance to be sought. Powers of observation are developed by training, and knowing what to look for and how to look for it are learned by experience.

General examination

Be alert to clues to respiratory disease which may be evident from the moment the patient is first seen (Fig. 2.1) or which become apparent during history taking. These include the rate and **character of breathing**, signs of respiratory distress such as **use of accessory muscles** of respiration (e.g. sternocleidomastoids), the **shape of the chest**, spine and shoulders and the character of any **cough**. **Hoarseness** of the voice may be a clue to recurrent laryngeal nerve damage by a carcinoma. **Stridor** or **wheeze** may be audible. Count the **respiratory rate** over a period of 30 seconds. The respiratory rate is best counted surreptitiously, perhaps while feeling the pulse, as patients tend to breath faster if they are aware that you are focusing on their breathing. Avoid proceeding directly to examination of the chest but first pause to look for signs in the hands such as **clubbing**, **tar staining** or **features of rheumatoid arthritis**. Signs of carbon dioxide retention include peripheral **vasodilatation** and **asterixis**, a flapping tremor detected by asking the patient to spread his or her fingers and cock the wrists back. It may be accentuated by applying gentle pressure against the patient's hands in this position. Count the **pulse rate** over 30 seconds and note any abnormalities in rhythm (e.g. atrial fibrillation) or character (e.g. a bounding pulse of carbon dioxide retention). Next examine the head and neck, particularly seeking signs of **cyanosis**, **anaemia** (pallor of conjunctiva), elevation of **jugular venous pressure** or **lymph node**

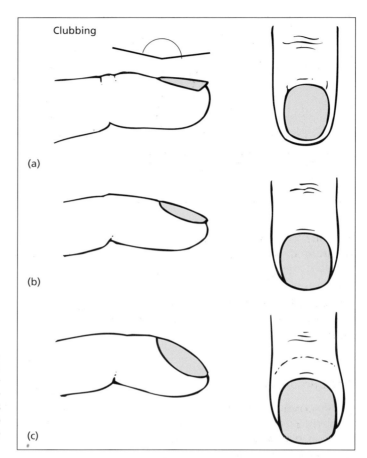

Figure 2.2 Clubbing. (a) Normal, showing the 'angle'. (b) Early clubbing; the angle is absent. (c) Advanced clubbing. The nail shows increased curvature in all directions, the angle is absent, the base of the nail is raised up by spongy tissue and the end of the digit is expanded.

enlargement. Be alert for uncommon signs such as **Horner's syndrome** (ptosis, meiosis, enophthalmos, anhydrosis) indicating damage to the sympathetic nerves by a tumour situated at the lung apex (see Chapter 13).

Clubbing

This is increased curvature of the nail with loss of the angle between the nail and nail bed (Fig. 2.2). It is a very important sign which is associated with a number of diseases (Table 2.3), most notably bronchial carcinoma and fibrotic lung disease, such as idiopathic pulmonary fibrosis and asbestosis. Advanced clubbing is sometimes associated with hypertrophic pulmonary osteoarthropathy in which

Answer to question in Fig. 2.1: (b) has airways obstruction—note the high position of the shoulders.

there is new bone formation in the subperiosteal region of the long bones of the arms and legs which is detectable on X-ray and is associated with pain and tenderness.

Cyanosis

This is a bluish discolouration of the skin and mucous membranes as a result of an excessive amount of reduced haemoglobin (usually >5 g/dL). **Central cyanosis** is best seen on the tip of the tongue and is the cardinal sign of hypoxaemia, although it is not a sensitive sign because it is not usually detectable until the oxygen saturation has fallen to well below 85%, corresponding to a Po_2 of <8 kPa (60 mmHg). Cyanosis is more difficult to detect if the patient is anaemic or has dark-coloured skin. Because of the poor sensitivity of cyanosis it is essential to measure oxygenation by

Table 2.3 Causes of clubbing.

Respiratory
- Neoplastic
  - Bronchial carcinoma
  - Mesothelioma
- Infections
  - Bronchiectasis
  - Cystic fibrosis
  - Chronic empyema
  - Lung abscess
- Fibrosis
  - Idiopathic pulmonary fibrosis
  - Asbestosis

Cardiac
- Bacterial endocarditis
- Cyanotic congenital heart disease
- Atrial myxoma

Gastrointestinal
- Hepatic cirrhosis
- Crohn's disease
- Coeliac disease

Congenital
- Idiopathic familial clubbing

oximetry or arterial blood gas sampling in patients at risk for hypoxaemia. **Peripheral cyanosis** may be caused by local circulatory slowing in the peripheries resulting in more complete extraction of oxygen from the blood (e.g. blue hands and ears in cold weather).

Jugular veins

Jugular veins are examined with the patient in a semi-reclining position with the trunk at an angle of about 45° from the horizontal. The head is turned slightly to the opposite side and fully supported so that the sternocleidomastoid muscles are relaxed. The jugular venous pulse is seen as a diffuse superficial pulsation of multiple wave form which is distinct from the carotid arterial pulse. The height of the pulse wave is measured from the top of the oscillating column of blood vertically to the sternal angle. The jugular venous pressure normally falls during inspiration. It is elevated in right heart failure which may occur as a result of pulmonary embolism or cor pulmonale

in COPD, for example. Other signs of right heart failure such as hepatomegaly and peripheral oedema may also be present.

Chest examination

Ask the patient to undress to the waist, and proceed to examine the chest in a methodical way using the techniques of inspection, palpation, percussion and auscultation.

Inspection

Look at the chest from the front, back and sides noting the overall **shape** and any **asymmetry**, **scars** or **skeletal abnormality**. The normal chest is flattened anteroposteriorly whereas the hyperinflated chest of COPD is barrel-shaped with an increased anteroposterior diameter. Watch the **movement** of the chest carefully as the patient breathes in and out. Diminished movement of one side of the chest is a clue to disease on that side. Overall movement is reduced if the lungs are hyperinflated (e.g. emphysema) or have reduced compliance (e.g. fibrosis). The costal margins normally move upwards and outwards in inspiration as the chest expands. In a chest which is already severely overinflated (e.g. COPD) there is sometimes paradoxical movement of the costal margins such that they are drawn inwards during inspiration: **costal margin paradox** (Fig. 2.3). The abdominal wall normally moves outwards on inspiration as the diaphragm descends. **Abdominal paradox**, in which the abdominal wall moves inwards during inspiration when the patient is supine, is a sign of diaphragm weakness.

Palpation

Chest movements during respiration may be more easily appreciated by placing the hands exactly symmetrically on either side of the upper sternum with the thumbs in the midline. The relative movement of the two hands and the separation of the thumbs reflect the overall movement of the chest and any asymmetry between the two sides. The position of the mediastinum is assessed by

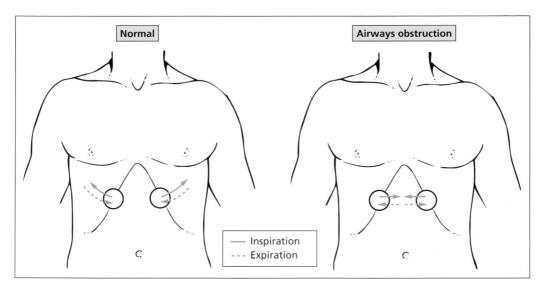

Figure 2.3 Movement of the costal margin. The arrows indicate the direction of movement in normal individuals and in those with airways obstruction (see text).

locating the **tracheal position** and the cardiac **apex beat**. Inserting a finger between the trachea and the sternocleidomastoid muscle on each side is a useful way of detecting any tracheal deviation. Running a finger gently up and down the trachea from the cricoid cartilage to the sternal notch may indicate the direction of the trachea as it enters the chest. Reduction in the **crico-sternal distance** is a sign of a hyperinflated chest. The apex beat is the most inferior and lateral point at which the cardiac impulse can be felt. The intercostal space in which the apex beat is felt should be counted down from the second intercostal space which is just below the sternal angle, and its location should also be related to landmarks such as the mid-clavicular or anterior axillary lines. It is normally located in the fifth left intercostal space in the mid-clavicular line. The mediastinum may be deviated towards or away from the side of disease. For example, fibrosis of the apex of the lung caused by previous tuberculosis may *pull* the trachea to that side, whereas a large pleural effusion or tension pneumothorax may *push* the trachea and apex beat away from the side of the lesion. **Tactile fremitus** refers to the ability to palpate vibrations set up by the voice in the large airways and transmitted to the chest wall. Ask the patient to say 'ninety-nine' or 'one, one, one' and palpate the vibrations, which are reduced in conditions such as pleural effusion or pleural thickening which muffle the transmission of the vibrations from the lung to the chest wall (Fig. 2.4). Consolidation of the lung may sometimes enhance transmission of the vibration.

Percussion

Percussion over normal air-filled lung produces a **resonant note** whereas percussion over solid organs such as the liver or heart produces a **dull note**. Abnormal dullness is found over areas of lung consolidation (e.g. lobar pneumonia) or fluid (e.g. pleural effusion). **Hyper-resonance** may be present in emphysema or over the area of a pneumo-thorax, although it is rarely a reliable sign. Percussion technique is important and requires practice. The resting finger should be placed flat against the chest wall in an intercostal space. The percussing finger should strike the dorsal surface of the middle phalanx and should be lifted clear after each percussion stroke. All areas should be percussed, paying particular attention to comparison between the two sides. When percussing the back of the

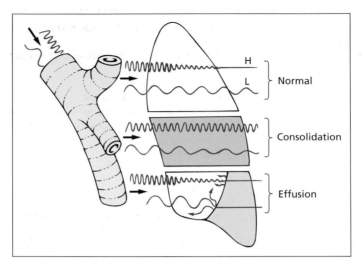

Figure 2.4 Summary of sound transmission in the lung. Sound is generated either by turbulence in the larynx and large airways, or by the voice. Both sources are a mixture of high- (H) and low- (L) pitched components. *Normal aerated lung* filters off the high-pitched component but transmits the low-pitched component quite well. This results in soft low-pitched breath sounds, well-conducted vocal resonance and easily palpable very-low-pitched sound (vocal fremitus). *Consolidated lung* transmits high-pitched sound well and filters off some of the lower pitched sound. This results in loud high-pitched breath sounds (bronchial breathing), high-pitched bleating vocal resonance (aegophony) and easy transmission of high-pitched consonants of speech (whispering pectoriloquy). *Pleural effusion* causes reduction in the transmission of all sound—probably because of reflection of sound waves at the air–fluid interface. Breath sounds are absent, vocal resonance much reduced and vocal fremitus is absent.

chest it is helpful to ask the patient to rotate his or her arms such that one elbow is placed on top of the other in order to bring the scapulae forward and out of the way.

Auscultation

Listen with the diaphragm or bell of the stethoscope to the **intensity** and **character** of the **breath sounds**, comparing both sides symmetrically, and note any **added sounds** (e.g. wheeze, crackles, pleural rub). The sources of audible sound in the lungs are turbulent airflow in the larynx and central airways and the voice. Reduction in the intensity of breath sounds (sometimes loosely referred to as reduced 'air entry') over an area of lung is an important sign which may, for example, indicate obstruction of a large bronchus preventing air from entering a lobe of the lung, or the presence of a pleural effusion reducing transmission of sound to the stethoscope. In normal individuals the **inspiratory phase** of respiration is usually longer than

the **expiratory phase**. Prolongation of the expiratory phase is a feature of airways obstruction and this is often accompanied by **wheeze (rhonchi)**— a high-pitched whistling or sighing sound. Diffuse wheeze is a feature of asthma or COPD. Wheeze localised to one side, or one area of the lung, suggests obstruction of a bronchus by a carcinoma or foreign body (e.g. inhaled peanut). **Crackles (crepitations)** may be loud and coarse or fine and high pitched, and may occur early or late in inspiration. It is thought that crackles are produced by the opening of previously closed bronchioles. The 'crackling' noise may be imitated by rolling a few hairs together close to the ear. Early crackles are sometimes heard at the beginning of inspiration in patients with COPD but these usually disappear when the patient is asked to cough. Persistent pan-inspiratory or late-inspiratory crackles are a feature of pulmonary oedema, lung fibrosis (e.g. idiopathic pulmonary fibrosis) or bronchiectasis. During inspiration, areas of lung open up in sequence according to their compliance (distensibility). In

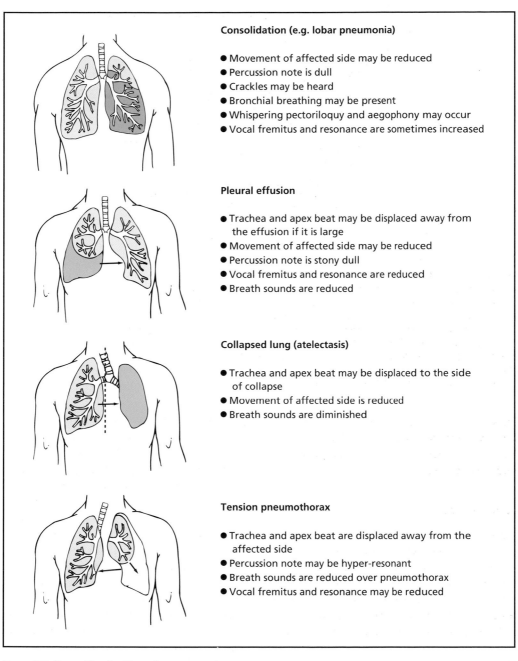

Consolidation (e.g. lobar pneumonia)

● Movement of affected side may be reduced
● Percussion note is dull
● Crackles may be heard
● Bronchial breathing may be present
● Whispering pectoriloquy and aegophony may occur
● Vocal fremitus and resonance are sometimes increased

Pleural effusion

● Trachea and apex beat may be displaced away from the effusion if it is large
● Movement of affected side may be reduced
● Percussion note is stony dull
● Vocal fremitus and resonance are reduced
● Breath sounds are reduced

Collapsed lung (atelectasis)

● Trachea and apex beat may be displaced to the side of collapse
● Movement of affected side is reduced
● Breath sounds are diminished

Tension pneumothorax

● Trachea and apex beat are displaced away from the affected side
● Percussion note may be hyper-resonant
● Breath sounds are reduced over pneumothorax
● Vocal fremitus and resonance may be reduced

Figure 2.5 Signs of localised lung disease.

airways obstruction there may be terminal airway closure during expiration, particularly in relatively compliant (floppy) parts of the lung damaged by emphysema. During inspiration air initially enters these areas more readily and crackles are probably produced by the opening of these airways early in inspiration. Coarse late-inspiratory crackles are particularly associated with diseases where there is reduced lung compliance (increased stiffness), which is to some extent patchily distributed. During inspiration, air first enters the more compliant parts of the lung and then enters the stiffer parts later in inspiration as elastic recoil forces build up in the stretching lung. **Pleural rubs** are 'creaking' sounds which are often quite localised and indicate roughening of the normally slippery pleural surfaces.

Vocal resonance is assessed by listening over the chest with the stethoscope as the patient says 'ninety-nine' or 'one, one, one' in much the same way as vocal fremitus is palpated. Normal aerated lung transmits the booming low-pitched components of speech and attenuates the high frequencies. Consolidated lung, however, filters off the low frequencies and transmits the higher frequencies so that speech takes on a bleating quality, **aegophony**. The facilitated transmission of high frequencies can be demonstrated by the clear transmission of whispering over consolidated lung, **whispering pectoriloquy**. The term 'bronchial breathing' refers to the harsher breath sounds normally heard over the trachea and main bronchi. It is also heard over areas of consolidated lung which conduct the higher frequency 'hiss' component from the larger airways.

Signs

See Fig. 2.5 for signs of localised lung disease. It is important to realise that major disease of the lungs may be present without any detectable physical signs and it is therefore essential to obtain a chest X-ray where there is good reason to suspect localised lung disease.

Keypoints

- The main respiratory symptoms are breathlessness, wheeze, cough, sputum, haemoptysis and chest pain.
- Haemoptysis is an important symptom which requires investigation as it may indicate lung cancer, laryngeal cancer, bronchitis or tuberculosis etc.
- Diminished movement of one side of the chest on inspiration is a clue to disease on that side.
- Major disease of the chest may be present without detectable signs, and tests (e.g. chest X-ray) are required where there is suspicion of lung disease.

Further reading

Irwin RS, Baumann MH, Bolser DC. Diagnosis and management of cough: American College of Chest Physicians: evidence-based clinical practice guidelines. Chest 2006; **129** (Suppl.): 1–292.

Naish JM, Read AE, Burns-Cox CJ. *The Clinical Apprentice*. Bristol: John Wright and Sons, 1978.

Ogilvie C. *Chamberlain's Symptoms and Signs in Clinical Medicine*. Bristol: John Wright and Sons, 1980.

Spiteri M, Cook D, Clarke S. Reliability of eliciting physical signs in examination of the chest. *Lancet* 1988; **i**: 873–5.

Chapter 3

Pulmonary function tests

Introduction

Pulmonary function tests are useful in defining respiratory disorders, in **quantifying** the severity of any deficit and in **monitoring** the course of the disease. Simple tests such as spirometry or measurement of peak expiratory flow (PEF) may be performed **in the consulting room, at the bedside** or by the patients themselves **at home**, whereas more complex tests require the facilities of a **lung function laboratory**. Normal values depend on the patient's height, age and sex, and tables and prediction equations are available for determining a patient's predicted normal value. The patient's test result may be compared with the mean reference value and standard deviation of results obtained in the healthy population or expressed as a percentage of the population's mean reference value. Pulmonary function tests should not be interpreted in isolation and should be considered in the context of all additional information concerning the patient.

Lung volumes (Fig. 3.1)

Tidal volume is the volume of air which enters and leaves the lungs during normal breathing. The volume of gas within the lungs at the end of a normal expiration is the **functional residual capacity**. The volume of gas in the lungs after a full inspiration is the **total lung capacity**. After a full expiration

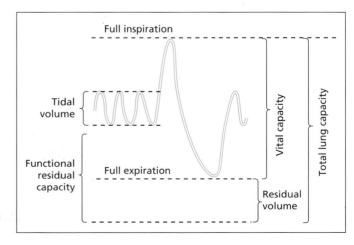

Figure 3.1 Total lung capacity and its subdivisions.

there is still some gas remaining in the lungs: the **residual volume**. **Vital capacity** (VC) is the volume of air expelled by a maximum expiration from a position of full inspiration. VC and its subdivisions can be measured directly by spirometry, whereas measurements of residual volume and total lung capacity require the use of gas dilution or plethysmography methods.

Spirometry

Spirometry measures changes in lung volume by recording changes in the volume of air exchanged through the airway opening (Fig. 3.2). Because residual volume cannot be exhaled, spirometry measurements are limited to VC and its subdivisions. One of the most useful techniques is to plot the volume of air exhaled from a patient's lungs against time during a forced expiratory manoeuvre: the **forced expiratory spirogram** (see Fig. 3.4).

Vital capacity

Vital capacity is the **volume of air expelled by a maximum expiration from a position of full inspiration**. It is often derived from a forced expiratory spirogram, with the patient exhaling with maximum effort, in which case it is referred to as the **forced vital capacity** (FVC). It may also be measured by a slow exhalation and this is sometimes referred to as the 'slow' VC. In normal individuals, slow VC and FVC are very similar but in patients with airways obstruction air trapping

occurs during forced expiration so that the FVC may be significantly smaller than the slow VC. The following circumstances may reduce VC:

- reduced lung compliance (e.g. lung fibrosis, loss of lung volume);
- chest deformity (e.g. kyphoscoliosis, ankylosing spondylitis);
- muscle weakness (e.g. myopathy, myasthenia gravis);
- airways obstruction (e.g. chronic obstructive pulmonary disease (COPD)—air trapping causes increased residual volume and reduced VC).

Forced expiratory volume in 1 second

Forced expiratory volume in 1 second (FEV_1) is the **volume of air expelled in the first second of a maximal forced expiration from a position of full inspiration**. It is reduced in any condition that reduces VC but it is particularly reduced when there is **diffuse airways obstruction**.

Forced expiratory volume in 1 second/forced vital capacity ratio

Normally, during a forced expiratory manoeuvre at least 75% of the air is expelled in the first second. In diffuse airways obstruction the FEV_1 is affected to a greater extent than the FVC and the ratio of FEV_1/FVC is reduced to below 0.75. This pattern is referred to as an **obstructive defect**. When lung volume is restricted by pulmonary fibrosis or rigidity of the chest wall for example,

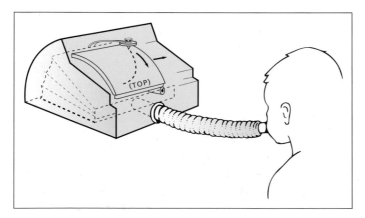

Figure 3.2 Schematic view of Vitalograph dry spirometer. The main components are a bellows and a moving record chart. An arm attached to the bellows carries a writing point which moves across the chart as air enters the bellows. As soon as the bellows moves, a microswitch is triggered and a motor causes the record chart to move steadily from left to right. The combination of lateral movement of the chart and forward movement of the writing point causes an oblique line to be inscribed upon the chart (see Fig. 3.4).

the VC is reduced and the FEV_1 is also reduced in proportion so that the FEV_1/FVC ratio is normal. This pattern of ventilatory impairment is referred to as a **restrictive defect**.

Maximal mid-expiratory flow

In addition to FEV_1 and FVC a number of other indices may be calculated from a forced expiratory spirogram. The maximal mid-expiratory flow **measured over the middle half of forced expiration** ($FEF_{25-75\%}$) reflects changes in the smaller **peripheral airways** whereas PEF and FEV_1 are predominantly influenced by diffuse changes of the medium-sized and larger airways.

Peak expiratory flow

PEF is the **maximum rate of airflow** which can be achieved **during a sudden forced expiration** from a position of full inspiration (Fig. 3.3). The best of three attempts is usually accepted as the peak flow rate. It is somewhat dependent on effort but is mainly determined by the calibre of the airways and is therefore an index of **diffuse airways**

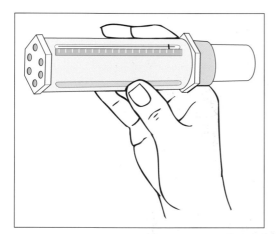

Figure 3.3 Measurement of PEF. The subject takes a *full inspiration*, applies the lips to the mouthpiece and makes a sudden maximal expiratory blast. A piston is pushed down the inside of the cylinder progressively exposing a slot in the top, until a position of rest is reached. The position of the piston is indicated by a marker and PEF read from a scale. It is customary to take the best of three properly performed attempts as the PEF.

obstruction. It is particularly useful in monitoring the course of asthma (see Chapter 11).

Flow–volume loop

The familiar spirometer trace plots volume against time (Fig. 3.4). Forced ventilatory manoeuvres may also be displayed by plotting **flow against volume in both expiration and inspiration**. This may be done using a pneumotachograph, which is a transducer comprising a small resistance to airflow through which the patient breathes. Pressure drop across this resistance is proportional to airflow. The pressure is converted to an electrical signal and displayed on an oscilloscope or plotter. The volume of air moved can be derived from electrical integration of the flow signal. A normal flow–volume loop is shown in Fig. 3.5. PEF is reached early in expiration from total lung capacity and is faster than peak inspiratory flow. There is a steady fall in expiratory flow as expiration progresses. The flow–volume loop is particularly used in assessing localised narrowing of the central airways as illustrated in Figs 3.6 and 3.7. Interpretation of the flow–volume loop may be difficult and the inspiratory portion is less reproducible than the expiratory portion, but flow–volume loops are useful in suggesting less common causes of **central airways obstruction** such as bilateral vocal cord palsy, tracheal tumours or tracheal compression by mediastinal disease. In practice, there is often difficulty in diagnosing these conditions, usually because the possibility is not considered and the patient is misdiagnosed as having asthma. Flow–volume loops or subtle changes on spirometry may point to the diagnosis and indicate the need for a definitive investigation such as bronchoscopy or computed tomography, for example.

Total lung capacity

Whereas VC and its subdivisions can be measured directly by spirometry, measurement of residual volume and total lung capacity require the use of **helium dilution** or **plethysmography** methods. In the dilution technique a gas of known helium

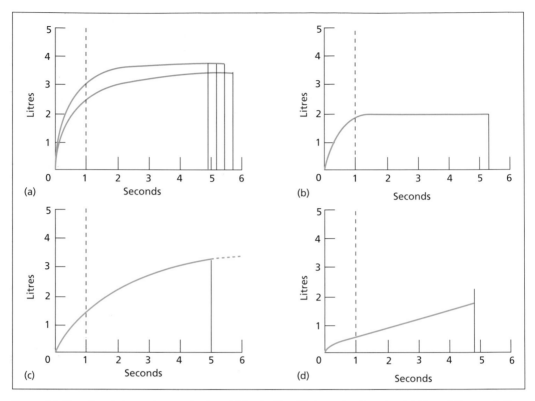

Figure 3.4 Forced expiratory spirogram tracing obtained with a Vitalograph spirometer. (a) *Normal.* Four expirations have been made. Three of these were true maximal forced expirations as indicated by their *reproducibility*. The forced expiratory volume in 1 second (FEV$_1$) is 3.2 L and the FVC is 3.8 L. The forced expiratory ratio (FEV$_1$/FVC) is 84%. (b) *Restrictive ventilatory defect.* Patient with pulmonary fibrosis. The FVC in this case was 2 L less than the predicted value for the subject. The FEV$_1$ is also reduced below the predicted value but it represents a large part of the FVC. The forced expiratory ratio is greater than 90%. (c) *Obstructive ventilatory defect.* The FEV$_1$ is much reduced. The rate of airflow is severely reduced as indicated by the reduced slope of the curve. Note that the forced expiratory time is increased—the patient is still blowing out at 5 seconds. The vital capacity has not been adequately recorded in this case because the patient did not continue the expiration after the chart stopped moving; he or she could have expired further. (This is a common technical error). (d) *Severe airways obstruction.* The FEV$_1$ is about 0.5 L. FVC is also reduced but not so strikingly as FEV$_1$. Forced expiratory ratio is 23%. Very low expiratory flow rate. This pattern of a very brief initial rapid phase followed by a straight line indicating little change in maximal flow rate with change in lung volume is sometimes associated with severe emphysema.

concentration is breathed through a closed circuit and the volume of gas in the lungs is calculated from a measure of the dilution of the helium, which, being an inert gas, is neither absorbed nor metabolised. This dilution method measures only gas in communication with the airways and tends to underestimate total lung capacity in patients with severe airways obstruction because of the presence of poorly ventilating bullae. The body plethysmograph is a large airtight box that allows the simultaneous determination of pressure–volume relationships in the thorax of a patient placed inside the box. When the plethysmograph is sealed, changes in lung volume are reflected by an increase in pressure within the plethysmograph. Plethysmography tends to overestimate total lung capacity because it measures all intrathoracic gas, including gas in bullae, cysts, stomach and oesophagus. The **chest X-ray** can be used to give a rough estimate of total lung capacity. In airways disease, residual volume is often increased as a manifestation of air trapping and total lung capacity increased as a

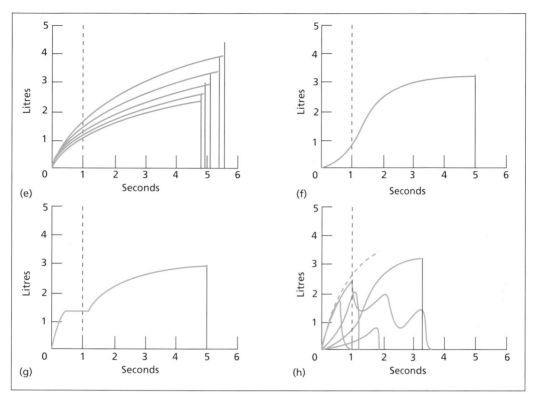

Figure 3.4 (*Continued*) (e) *Airways obstruction and bronchial hyper-reactivity.* Five expirations have been made. FEV_1 and FVC become lower with each expiration. Patient with asthma. These features suggest poor control of asthma and liability to severe attacks. (f) *A non-maximal expiration.* Compare with (a). In a true forced expiration the steepest part of the curve always occurs at the beginning of expiration which is not the case in (f). A falsely low FEV_1 and forced expiratory ratio are obtained. Usually the patient has not understood what is required or is unable to coordinate his or her actions. Some patients wish to appear worse than they really are. This pattern is unlikely to be mistaken for a true forced expiration because of its shape and because it cannot be reproduced repeatedly. (g) *Escape of air* from the nose or lips during expiration. (h) *Inability to perform the manoeuvre.* Five attempts have been made. In some the patient has breathed in and out. Other attempts are either not maximal forced expirations or are unfinished. Bizarre patterns such as this are often seen in patients with psychogenic breathlessness and in the elderly and demented. Even with poor cooperation it is often possible to obtain useful information. In the example shown (h), significant airways obstruction can be excluded because of the steep slope of at least two of the expirations which follow an identical course and show appropriate curvature (dotted line) and the FVC can be estimated as not less than 3.2 L. The pattern seen in large airways obstruction is shown in Fig. 3.6.

manifestation of hyperinflation. Total lung capacity is reduced in restrictive lung disease.

Transfer factor for carbon monoxide

The **rate at which gas passes from the alveoli to the bloodstream** can be measured using a low concentration of carbon monoxide. The transfer of carbon monoxide across the alveolar capillary membrane is similar to that of oxygen. Oxygen diffusion is difficult to measure because transport stops when haemoglobin becomes saturated. At one time it was thought that the main factor limiting gas exchange in disease was the ability of gases to diffuse across the alveolar capillary membrane. This led to the concept of **diffusing capacity** for carbon monoxide ($D_L CO$). It was later realised that

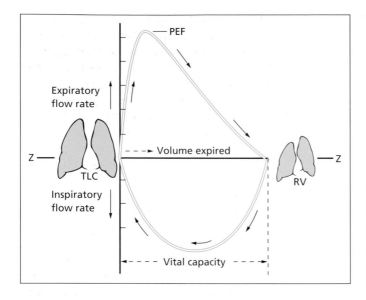

Figure 3.5 The flow–volume loop. Airflow is represented on the vertical axis and lung volume on the horizontal axis. The line Z–Z represents zero flow. Expiratory flow appears above the line; inspiratory flow below. PEF, peak expiratory flow; RV, residual volume; TLC, total lung capacity.

many other factors (e.g. ventilation/perfusion matching) influenced gas transfer and the expression was renamed **transfer factor** ($T_L\text{CO}$). The **transfer coefficient** ($K\text{CO}$) is an expression of gas transfer standardised for the alveolar volume (V_A).

Single-breath method (Fig. 3.8)

The patient inspires a gas mixture of helium and carbon monoxide, holds the breath for 10 seconds and then breathes out. An initial volume equivalent to the deadspace is discarded and then a sample of the expired gas is collected and analysed for alveolar concentrations of helium and carbon monoxide. The change in concentration of helium between the inspired and alveolar sample is the result of gas dilution and gives a measurement of the alveolar gas volume (V_A). The expired concentration of carbon monoxide is also lower than the inspired level but the fall is proportionately greater than in the case of helium because some of the carbon monoxide has been absorbed into the bloodstream. The rate of uptake of carbon monoxide can then be calculated as the uptake of carbon monoxide per minute per unit of partial pressure of carbon monoxide (mmol/min/kPa), or as the carbon monoxide transfer coefficient ($K\text{CO}$) which is the $T_L\text{CO}$ standardised for V_A.

Steady-state method

The patient breathes air containing a known low concentration of carbon monoxide from a Douglas bag and expired air is collected in another Douglas bag over a timed period of some minutes. The rate of carbon monoxide transfer can be calculated from the difference between inspired and expired concentrations. A mean alveolar carbon monoxide level can be calculated by estimating a deadspace ventilation for carbon dioxide and assuming that this same volume was filled with unchanged inspired carbon monoxide mixture. The shortfall in expired carbon monoxide must then be entirely brought about by a lower concentration in the alveolar fraction which can be calculated, and the transfer of carbon monoxide can be derived.

Although $T_L\text{CO}$ and $K\text{CO}$ are influenced by many factors (e.g. ventilation/perfusion (V/Q) imbalance, area of alveolar membrane, haemoglobin level) they are very useful measurements in clinical practice. A reduced $T_L\text{CO}$ is a strong indicator of a **parenchymal lung disorder** involving the alveoli or their blood supply. It is reduced, for example, in emphysema, fibrotic lung disease (e.g. idiopathic pulmonary fibrosis) and pulmonary embolism. It may be increased in asthma (probably because of improved distribution of ventilation and perfusion),

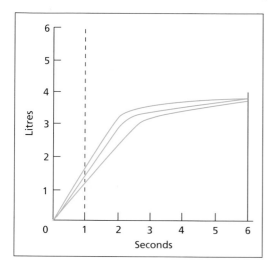

Figure 3.6 Large (central) airways obstruction. Typical tracing obtained with a Vitalograph spirometer. The subject has made three maximal forced expirations. Each shows a striking straight section which then changes relatively abruptly, at about the same volume, to follow the expected curve of the forced expiratory spirogram. The straight section is not as reproducible as a normal spirogram. A 'family' of similar tracings is thus obtained, each with straight and curved sections. Explanation: over the straight section, flow is limited by the fixed intrathoracic localised obstruction. This is little influenced by lung recoil so the critical flow is similar during expiration and the spirogram appears straight. A lung volume is eventually reached where maximum flow is even lower than that permitted by the central obstruction. The ordinary forced expiratory spirogram is described after this point. In the example shown there must be an element of diffuse airways obstruction, as forced expiratory time is somewhat prolonged (see Fig. 3.4c).

polycythaemia and alveolar haemorrhage (because extravasated blood binds carbon monoxide). Adjusting the $T_{L}CO$ for alveolar volume, giving the transfer coefficient (KCO), is useful in assessing if the reduced transfer factor is a result of a loss of surface area for diffusion. For example, a patient who has had one lung removed will have a reduced $T_{L}CO$ but a normal KCO if the remaining lung is normal.

Respiratory muscle function tests

Weakness of the respiratory muscles causes a **restrictive ventilatory defect** with reduced total lung capacity and VC. Comparison of the VC in the erect and supine position is useful because the pressure of the abdominal contents on a weak diaphragm typically causes a fall of >30% in the **supine VC**. **Chest X-ray** often shows small lung fields with basal atelectasis and high hemidiaphragms. **Fluoroscopy screening** may show paradoxical upward movement of a weakened diaphragm during inspiration. When there is severe respiratory muscle weakness ventilatory failure develops with **hypercapnia**. Global respiratory muscle function may be assessed by measuring **mouth pressures**. Maximum inspiratory mouth pressure, P_I **max**, is measured during maximum inspiratory effort from residual volume against an obstructed airway using a mouthpiece and transducer device, and maximum expiratory mouth pressure, P_E **max**, is measured during a maximal expiratory effort from total lung capacity. The maximum **transdiaphragmatic pressure** generated during contraction can be measured in specialist laboratories using balloon catheters in the oesophagus and stomach.

Arterial blood gases

A **sample of arterial blood** may be obtained from any artery but the **radial artery** at the wrist or the **brachial artery** in the antecubital fossa are the sites most commonly used. Arterial puncture may be a painful procedure if there is difficulty in entering the artery quickly and directly so that **local anaesthetic** (e.g. 1% lidocaine (lignocaine)) may be helpful. The blood enters the **heparinised needle** and syringe under its own pressure with a pulsatile action. The syringe containing the arterial blood is capped, placed in **ice** and analysed in the laboratory within 30 minutes of sampling.

The normal range for P_{O_2} in healthy young adults is about 11–14 kPa (83–105 mmHg), and for P_{CO_2} about 4.5–6 kPa (34–45 mmHg). P_{CO_2} is an index of alveolar ventilation and rises if there is a decrease in ventilation. P_{O_2} falls reciprocally with the increase in P_{CO_2} when there is alveolar underventilation but it also falls when there is V/Q mismatch, which is a common disturbance in lung disease.

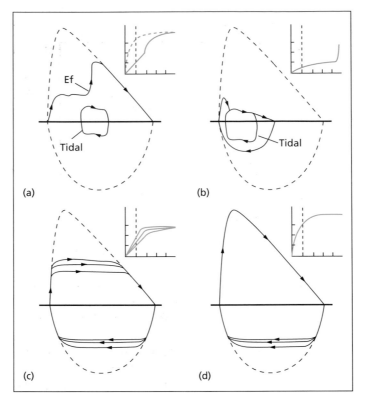

Figure 3.7 Further flow–volume loops. The dotted outline represents a typical normal loop. The small graphs show the appearances of a forced expiration on a Vitalograph spirometer (as in Fig. 3.4). (a) *Demonstration of maximum flow.* A normal individual makes an unhurried expiration from full inspiration and then about halfway through the vital capacity, a maximal expiratory effort (Ef) is made. The flow–volume tracing rejoins the maximum flow–volume curve which describes the highest flow which can be achieved at that lung volume. Also shown in (a) is the flow–volume loop of typical tidal breathing. At the resting lung volume there is an abundant reserve of both inspiratory and expiratory flow available. (b) *Very severe airways obstruction* in an individual with emphysema. Maximum expiratory flow is very severely reduced. There is a brief peak (probably caused by airway collapse) after which flow falls very slowly. Also shown in (b) is a loop representing quiet tidal breathing. It is clear that every expiration is limited by maximum flow. Expiratory wheezing or purse lip breathing would be expected. There is some inspiratory reserve of flow but hardly any expiratory reserve. Ventilation could be increased slightly by adopting an even higher lung volume and by speeding up inspiration. (c) *Fixed intrathoracic large airways obstruction:* for example, tracheal compression by a mediastinal tumour. Here the peak inspiratory and expiratory flows have been truncated in a characteristic pattern. (d) *Variable extrathoracic obstruction.* Severe extrathoracic obstruction results in inspiratory collapse of the airway below the obstruction (but still outside the thorax). In this example expiration is normal, and this suggests a variable check-valve mechanism such as might be caused by bilateral vocal cord paralysis.

Respiratory failure

Respiratory failure is a clinical term used to describe failure to maintain oxygenation (usually taken as an arbitrary cut-off point of Po_2 8.0 kPa (60 mmHg)).

- *Type I respiratory failure* is hypoxaemia in the absence of hypercapnia and usually indicates a severe disturbance of V/Q relationships in the lungs. This pattern is seen in many conditions including pulmonary oedema, asthma, pulmonary embolism and lung fibrosis (Table 3.1).
- *Type II respiratory failure* is hypoxaemia with hypercapnia and indicates alveolar hypoventilation. This may occur from lack of neuromuscular control

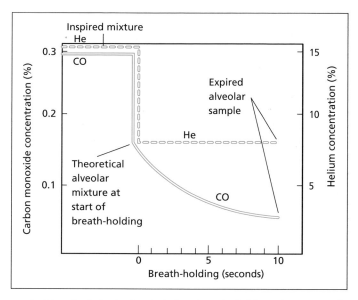

Figure 3.8 Measurement of transfer factor by the single-breath method. Schematic representation of the helium and carbon monoxide concentrations in the inspired mixture and in alveolar air during breath holding.

of ventilation (e.g. sedative overdose, cerebrovascular disease, myopathy) or from lung disease (e.g. COPD).

Oximetry

Oxygen saturation can be measured non-invasively and continuously using a pulse oximeter. Oxygenated blood appears red whereas reduced blood appears blue (clinical sign of cyanosis). An oximeter measures the ratio of oxygenated to total haemoglobin in arterial blood using a probe placed on a finger or ear lobe, which comprises two light-emitting diodes—one red and one infrared—and a detector. The light absorbed varies with each pulse, and measurement of light absorption at two points of the pulse wave allows the oxygen saturation of arterial blood to be determined. The accuracy of measurement is reduced if there is reduced arterial pulsation (e.g. low-output cardiac states) or increased venous pulsation (e.g. tricuspid regurgitation, venous congestion). Skin pigmentation or use of nail varnish may interfere with light transmission. Oximetry is also inaccurate in the presence of carboxyhaemoglobin (e.g. in carbon monoxide poisoning) which the oximeter detects as oxyhaemoglobin. The

Table 3.1 Examples of arterial gas measurements in various conditions.

P_{O_2}	P_{CO_2}	A–a gradient	
kPa (mmHg)	kPa (mmHg)	kPa (mmHg)	Diagnosis
13 (98)	5 (38)	2 (15)	Normal
8 (60)	10 (75)	2 (15)	Sedative overdose Reduced ventilation Type II respiratory failure
6 (45)	4 (30)	10 (75)	Fibrotic lung disease V/Q mismatch Type I respiratory failure
15 (112)	3 (23)	2 (15)	Psychogenic hyperventilation
18 (135)	5 (38)	?	Patient not breathing air as $P_{O_2} + P_{CO_2} > 20$ kPa

A–a gradient: the alveolar to arterial gradient $= P_{I_{O_2}} - (P_{O_2} + P_{CO_2})$ (see Chapter 1).

relationship of P_{O_2} to oxygen saturation is described by the **oxyhaemoglobin dissociation curve** (see Fig. 1.5). This curve is sigma-shaped so that oxygen saturation is closely related to P_{O_2} only over a short range of about 3–7 kPa. Above this level the dissociation curve begins to plateau and there is only a small increase in oxygen saturation as the P_{O_2} rises. Oximetry can reduce the need for arterial puncture, but arterial blood gas analysis is necessary to determine accurately the P_{O_2} on the plateau part of the oxyhaemoglobin dissociation curve, to measure carbon dioxide level and to assess acid–base status.

Acid–base balance

The three variables principally involved in acid–base balance in the body are **hydrogen ion concentration ([H$^+$])**, P_{CO_2} and **bicarbonate [HCO$_3^-$]**. [H$^+$] is generally expressed as pH which is the negative logarithm of [H$^+$]. These variables are directly related to each other in terms of the Henderson–Hasselbalch equation [H$^+$]$\propto$ P_{CO_2}/[HCO$_3^-$]. There is a direct linear relationship between P_{CO_2} and [H$^+$]. Bicarbonate concentration can be calculated if P_{CO_2} and pH are known or it can be measured directly: the **actual bicarbonate** concentration. **Standard bicarbonate** is a calculated value indicating what the bicarbonate would be at a standard P_{CO_2} of 5.3 kPa (40 mmHg). The **base excess** is a further parameter of the buffering capacity of the blood which recognises the fact that there are other buffers apart from bicarbonate in the blood. Changes in pH which are caused primarily by an alteration in P_{CO_2} are termed **respiratory**, and are determined by **alveolar ventilation**. Changes in pH which are brought about by changes in bicarbonate concentration are termed **metabolic**. The renal tubules modulate bicarbonate concentration in response to the prevailing P_{CO_2} but this is a slow process.

- *Acute respiratory acidosis*: **pH reduced, P_{CO_2} raised, bicarbonate normal.** A reduction in alveolar ventilation causes an increase in arterial P_{CO_2}. The pH falls in relation to the P_{CO_2}. In the short term there is insufficient time for renal compensation by reabsorption of bicarbonate so that the bicarbonate concentration remains almost unchanged. This pattern is seen where there is acute hypoventilation, for example obstruction of

the airway, overdose of sedative drugs or acute neurological damage.

- *Respiratory alkalosis*: **pH raised, P_{CO_2} reduced, bicarbonate normal.** Alveolar hyperventilation causes a fall in P_{CO_2} and a corresponding rise in pH. Bicarbonate concentration is virtually unchanged unless there is a longstanding respiratory alkalosis which is unusual. This pattern is seen in any form of acute hyperventilation, for example anxiety-related hyperventilation, salicylate poisoning, acute asthma.

- *Metabolic acidosis*: **pH reduced, P_{CO_2} reduced, bicarbonate reduced.** The primary disturbance is generally an increase in acid. This has an effect on the equilibrium H$^+$ + HCO$_3^-$ $\leftrightarrow$ H$_2$O + CO$_2$ pushing it to the right. The carbon dioxide produced is removed by increased ventilation and the net result is a lowering of plasma bicarbonate. In practice the fall in pH causes respiratory stimulation so that carbon dioxide is promptly blown off. This respiratory compensation is an inevitable accompaniment of metabolic acidosis—acute and chronic—unless there is some other factor limiting ventilatory function or responsiveness. This pattern is seen in diabetic ketoacidosis, renal tubular acidosis and acute circulatory failure and other forms of lactic acidosis.

- *Metabolic alkalosis*: **pH raised, P_{CO_2} normal or slightly raised, bicarbonate raised.** An increase in bicarbonate concentration causes a rise in pH. The compensatory fall in alveolar ventilation is usually slight, therefore P_{CO_2} usually increases a little. This pattern is seen where there has been administration of excessive alkali, loss of acid through vomiting, or reabsorption of bicarbonate (e.g. in hypokalaemia).

- *Chronic respiratory acidosis*: **pH normal or slightly reduced, P_{CO_2} raised, bicarbonate raised.** If alveolar hypoventilation is sustained for some days, renal tubular reabsorption of bicarbonate will achieve significant elevation of plasma bicarbonate level tending to correct the acidosis (chronic compensated respiratory acidosis). This pattern is seen in any cause of sustained hypoventilation, for example COPD, chronic neuromuscular disease.

- *Mixed disturbances*: **mixed respiratory and metabolic disturbances** are common and there are usually a number of possible explanations, therefore it is essential to consider all the clinical details before

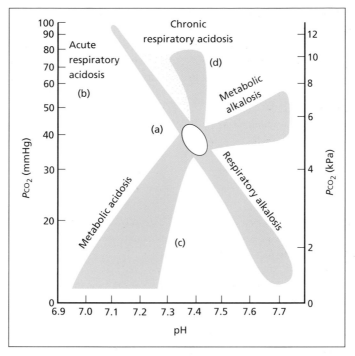

Figure 3.9 Acid–base disturbances. The oval indicates the normal position. The shaded areas indicate the direction of observed 'pure' or uncomplicated disturbances of acid–base balance. Bicarbonate levels are omitted for clarity. Letters (a)–(d) are referred to in the text (see Mixed disturbances).

interpreting the acid–base data. Figure 3.9 shows the situations that may arise in complex acid–base disturbances. For example, point (a) in Fig. 3.9 (low pH, normal P_{CO_2}, low bicarbonate) indicates a mixed metabolic and respiratory acidosis. This could arise in a patient with acute pulmonary oedema who is hypoxaemic with low cardiac output. The metabolic acidosis results from lactic acidosis and the patient's ability to hyperventilate is compromised. The same situation could arise in a totally different set of clinical circumstances (e.g. a patient in renal failure given a narcotic sedative suppressing ventilatory response to acidosis) so that acid–base data have limited diagnostic potential considered alone. Point (b) could represent the situation soon after a cardiac arrest where severe lactic acidosis exists and ventilation has been insufficient. Point (c) could represent the situation in severe aspirin poisoning where aspirin-induced hyperventilation has been complicated by aspirin-induced metabolic acidosis. Point (d) could represent

the situation in an individual with chronic hypercapnia as a result of COPD who is stimulated to increase ventilation by a pulmonary embolism.

Keypoints

- A reduced FEV₁/VC ratio indicates airways obstruction, for example asthma, COPD.
- A reduced K_{CO} and $T_{L}CO$ indicates disease of the lung parenchyma or its blood supply for example emphysema, lung fibrosis, pulmonary embolism.
- Type 1 respiratory failure is hypoxaemia without hypercapnia and occurs in asthma, pulmonary oedema, pulmonary embolism and lung fibrosis.
- Type 2 respiratory failure is hypoxaemia with hypercapnia and indicates hypoventilation which occurs in COPD, sedative overdosage or neuromuscular disease.

FEV₁: forced expiratory volume in one second; VC: vital capacity

$T_{L}CO$: transfer factor for carbon monoxide; K_{CO}: transfer coefficient

COPD: chronic obstructive pulmonary disease

Further reading

Cotes JE. *Lung Function: Assessment and Application in Medicine*. Oxford: Blackwell Scientific Publications, 1993.

Flenley DC. Interpretation of blood-gas and acid–base data. *Br J Hosp Med* 1978; **20**: 384–94.

Gibson GJ. *Clinical Tests of Respiratory Function*. Oxford: Chapman and Hall, 1996.

Gibson GJ. Measurement of respiratory muscle strength. *Respir Med* 1995; **89**: 529–35.

Hanning CD, Alexander-Williams JM. Pulse oximetry: a practical review. *BMJ* 1995; **311**: 367–70.

Chapter 4

Radiology of the chest

Chest X-ray

The chest X-ray has a key role in the investigation of respiratory disease. The standard view is the erect, **postero-anterior (PA) chest X-ray** taken at full inspiration with the X-ray beam passing from back to front. A **lateral X-ray** gives a better view of lesions lying behind the heart or diaphragm, which may not be visible on a PA X-ray, and allows abnormalities to be viewed in a further dimension. Supine and **antero-posterior (AP) views** are usually taken at the bedside using mobile equipment in patients who are too ill to be brought to the X-ray department. AP films are less satisfactory in defining many abnormalities, producing magnification of the cardiac outline, for example.

The main landmarks of the normal chest X-ray are shown in Figs 4.1 and 4.2. X-rays should be examined both close up and from a short distance on a viewing box or computer screen in an area with reduced background lighting. It is important to confirm the name and date on the X-ray and to check the technical quality of the film. Symmetry between the medial end of both clavicles and the thoracic spine confirms that the film has been taken without any rotation artefact. If the film has been taken in full inspiration the right hemidiaphragm is normally intersected by the anterior part of the sixth rib. The vertebral bodies are usually visible through the cardiac shadow if the X-ray

exposure is satisfactory. It is helpful to examine the film systematically to avoid missing useful information. The shape and bony structures of the chest wall should be surveyed and the position of the hemidiaphragms and trachea noted. The shape and size of the heart and the appearances of the mediastinum and hilar shadows are examined. The size, shape and disposition of the vascular shadows are noted and the pattern of the lung markings in different zones carefully compared. It is advisable to focus attention on areas of the chest X-ray where lesions are commonly missed such as the lung apices, hila and the area behind the heart. Any abnormality detected should be analysed in detail and interpreted in the context of all clinical information. It is often helpful to obtain previous X-rays or to monitor the evolution of abnormalities over time on follow-up X-rays. Some of the radiological features of the major lung diseases are shown in individual chapters. In some circumstances chest X-ray abnormalities follow a specific pattern which allows a differential diagnosis to be outlined.

Abnormal features

Collapse

Obstruction of a bronchus by a carcinoma, foreign body (e.g. inhaled peanut) or mucus plug causes

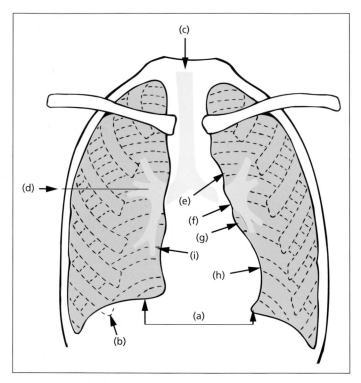

Figure 4.1 Diagram of chest X-ray (PA view). The right hemidiaphragm is 1–3 cm higher than the left (a) and on full inspiration it is intersected by the shadow of the anterior part of the sixth rib (b). The trachea (c) is vertical and central or very slightly to the right. The horizontal fissure (d) is found in the position shown, or slightly lower and should be truly horizontal. It is a very valuable marker of change in volume of any part of the right lung. The left border of the cardiac shadow comprises: (e) aorta; (f) pulmonary artery; (g) concavity overlying the left atrial appendage; (h) left ventricle. The right border of the cardiac shadow normally overlies the right atrium (i) and above that the superior vena cava.

loss of aeration with '**loss of volume**' and collapse of the lung distal to the obstruction. Collapse of each individual lobe of the lung produces its own particular appearance on chest X-ray (Figs 4.3 and 4.4) with **shift of landmarks** such as the mediastinum resulting from loss of volume. Obstruction of a main bronchus usually causes obvious asymmetry (Fig. 4.5). **Compensatory expansion** of other lobes may result in increased transradiency of adjacent areas of the lung. In right middle lobe collapse there may be little to see on a PA X-ray apart from lack of definition of the right heart border. This is a useful sign which helps to distinguish it from lower lobe collapse where the right border of the heart remains clearly defined. Left lower lobe collapse is manifest as a triangular area of increased density behind the heart shadow, often with a shift of the heart shadow to the left and increased transradiency of the left hemithorax because of compensatory expansion of the left upper lobe (Fig. 4.4). Collapse is a sinister sign often indicating an obstructing carcinoma which may be confirmed by bronchoscopy.

Consolidation

Air in the lungs appears black on X-ray. Consolidation appears as **areas of opacification** sometimes conforming to the outline of a lobe or segment of lung in which the air has been replaced by an inflammatory exudate (e.g. pneumonia), fluid (e.g. pulmonary oedema), blood (e.g. pulmonary

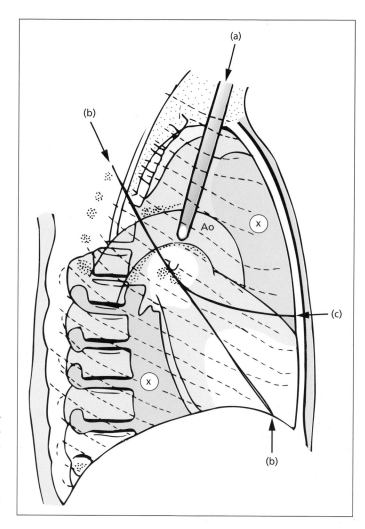

Figure 4.2 Diagram of chest X-ray (lateral view). (a) Trachea. (b) Oblique fissure. (c) Horizontal fissure. It is useful to note that in a normal lateral view the radiodensity of the lung field above and in front of the cardiac shadow is about the same as that below and behind (x). Ao, aorta.

haemorrhage) or tumour (e.g. alveolar cell carcinoma). Bronchi containing air passing through the consolidated lung are sometimes clearly visible as black tubes of air against the white background of the consolidated lung: **air bronchograms** (see Fig. 18.2, p. 193). Structures such as the heart, mediastinum and diaphragm are usually clearly outlined as a silhouette on an X-ray because of the contrast between the blackness of aerated lung and the whiteness of these structures. When there is abnormal shadowing in the lung adjacent to these structures there is loss of the sharp outline, and this is often referred to as the **silhouette sign**.

Pulmonary masses (Table 4.1, Fig. 4.6)

Various descriptive terms such as 'rounded opacity', 'nodule' or 'coin lesion' are used to refer to pulmonary masses. Carcinoma of the lung is the most important cause of a mass on chest X-ray but several other diseases may cause a similar appearance. Features such as **cavitation**, **calcification**, **rate of growth**, the presence of **associated abnormalities** (e.g. lymph node enlargement) and whether the lesion is **solitary** or whether **multiple** lesions are present, may provide clues to diagnosis. However, these features are often not reliable indicators of aetiology, and the X-ray appearances must be

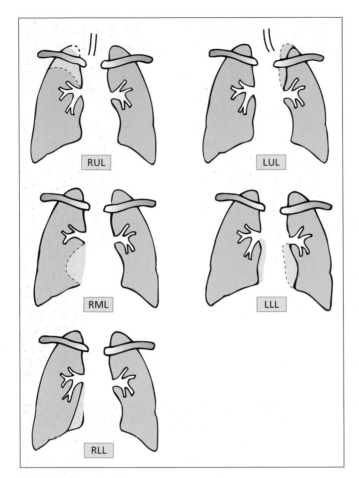

Figure 4.3 Radiographic patterns of lobar collapse. Collapsed lobes occupy a surprisingly small volume and are commonly overlooked on the chest X-ray. Helpful information may be provided by the position of the trachea, the hilar vascular shadows and the horizontal fissure. LLL, left lower lobe; LUL, left upper lobe; RLL, right lower lobe; RML, right middle lobe; RUL, right upper lobe.

interpreted in the context of all the clinical information. Further investigations such as computed tomography (CT) and biopsy (bronchoscopic, percutaneous, surgical) are often necessary.

Cavitation

Cavitation is the presence of an area of radiolucency within a mass lesion. It is a feature of **bronchial carcinoma** (particularly squamous carcinoma) (Fig. 4.7), **tuberculosis**, **lung abscess**, **pulmonary infarcts**, **Wegener's granulomatosis** (see p. 179) and some **pneumonias** (e.g. *Staphylococcus aureus*, *Klebsiella pneumoniae*).

Fibrosis

Localised fibrosis produces **streaky shadows** with evidence of **traction** upon neighbouring structures.

Upper lobe fibrosis causes traction upon the trachea and elevation of the hilar vascular shadows. Generalised interstitial fibrosis produces a hazy shadowing with a **fine reticular (net-like)** or **nodular pattern** (see Chapter 14). Advanced interstitial fibrosis results in a honeycomb pattern with diffuse opacification containing multiple circular translucencies a few millimetres in diameter.

Mediastinal masses

Metastatic tumour or lymphomatous involvement of the mediastinal lymph nodes are the most common causes of mediastinal masses but there are a number of other diseases which may cause mediastinal masses (Fig. 4.8). Thymic tumours, thyroid masses and dermoid cysts are most commonly situated in the anterior mediastinum whereas

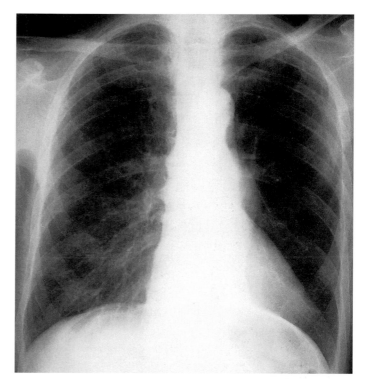

Figure 4.4 Left lower lobe collapse. The left lower lobe has collapsed medially and posteriorly and appears as a dense white triangular area behind the heart close to the mediastinum. The remainder of the left lung appears hyperlucent because of compensatory expansion. Bronchoscopy showed an adenocarcinoma occluding the left lower lobe bronchus.

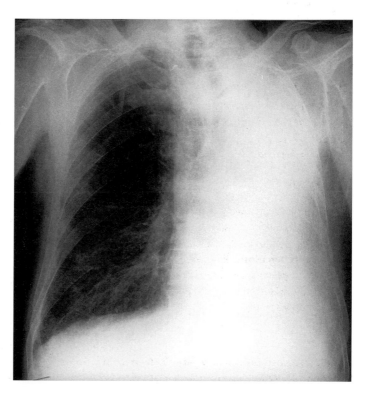

Figure 4.5 Left lung collapse. There is complete opacification of the left hemithorax with shift of the mediastinum to the left. Bronchoscopy showed a small-cell carcinoma occluding the left main bronchus.

neural lesions (e.g. neurofibroma) and oesophageal cysts are often situated posteriorly. Aneurysmal enlargement of the aorta or ventricle may produce masses in the middle compartment of the mediastinum. CT scans are helpful in delineating the anatomy of mediastinal lesions. Thoracotomy with surgical excision is often necessary.

Ultrasonography of the chest

Normal air-filled lung does not transmit high-frequency sound waves so that ultrasonography is not useful in assessing disease of lung parenchyma. It may be helpful in assessing lesions of the pleura and is particularly useful for localising loculated pleural effusions.

Computed tomography

CT scanning uses a technique of multiple projection with reconstruction of the image from X-ray detectors by a computer so that structures can be displayed in cross-section. A number of different techniques can be used depending on the area of interest, and interpretation of CT images will normally be carried out by an expert radiologist. CT scanning is particularly useful in providing a detailed cross-sectional image of mediastinal disease which is often difficult to assess on plain chest X-ray. Figure 4.9 shows the principal mediastinal structures with horizontal lines indicating the levels of the CT sections illustrated diagrammatically in Fig. 4.10. CT scanning is particularly important in the staging of the lung cancer (see Chapter 13), and has replaced bronchography (instillation of radiocontrast dye into the bronchial tree) in detecting and determining the extent of bronchiectasis (see Chapter 9). High-resolution CT scans are much more sensitive than plain X-ray in assessing the lung parenchyma and

Table 4.1 Causes of pulmonary masses.

Neoplastic
Primary bronchial carcinoma
Metastatic carcinoma
Benign tumours (hamartoma)
Non-neoplastic
Tuberculoma
Lung abscess
Hydatid cyst
Pulmonary infarct
Arteriovenous malformation
Encysted interlobar effusion –('pseudotumour')
Rheumatoid nodule

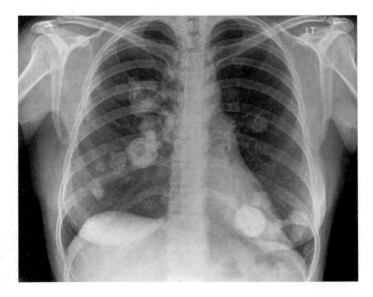

Figure 4.6 Chest X-ray showing multiple partially calcified rounded masses in both lungs due to benign chondromas.

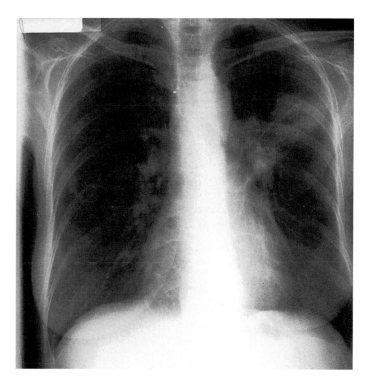

Figure 4.7 A cavitating lesion in the left upper lobe. A cavity appears as an area of radiolucency (black) within an opacity (white). Sputum cytology showed cells from a squamous carcinoma. CT showed left hilar and sub-carinal lymphadenopathy.

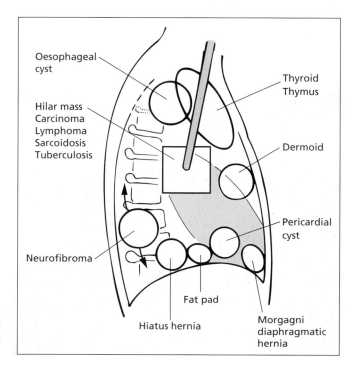

Figure 4.8 Mediastinal masses. Diagram of lateral view of the chest, indicating the sites favoured by some of the more common mediastinal masses.

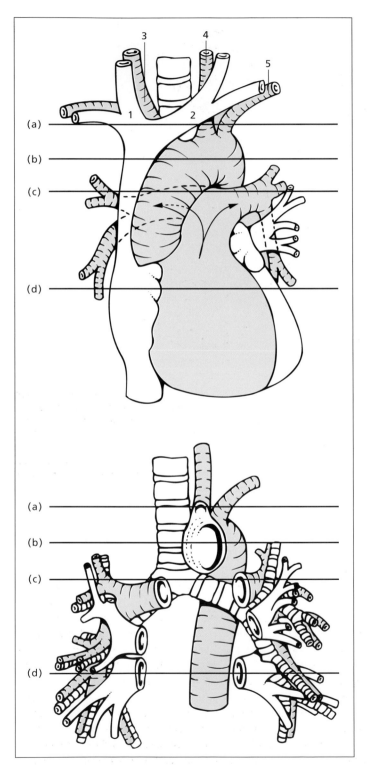

Figure 4.9 Mediastinal structures.
Principal blood vessels and airways.
Top: Heart and major blood vessels showing the aorta curling over the bifurcation of the pulmonary trunk into left and right pulmonary arteries (arrows). The horizontal lines (a)–(d) indicate the levels of the CT sections illustrated in Fig. 4.10. 1, right brachiocephalic vein; 2, left brachiocephalic vein; 3, innominate or brachiocephalic artery; 4, left common carotid artery; 5, left subclavian artery.
Bottom: Structures with the heart removed. The aorta curls over the left main bronchus which lies behind the left pulmonary artery. Pulmonary arteries are shown shaded, pulmonary veins unshaded and bronchi are shown striped. In general the arteries loop downwards, like a handlebar moustache; veins radiate towards a lower common destination—the left atrium. The veins are applied to the front of the arteries and bronchi and take a slightly different path to the respective lung segments. On the right, the order of structures from front to back is vein–artery–bronchus; on the left, the pulmonary artery loops over the left upper lobe bronchus and descends behind so that the order is vein–bronchus–artery.

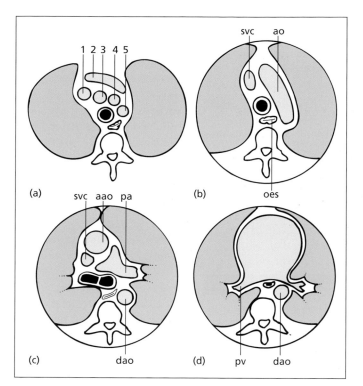

Figure 4.10 Principal mediastinal structures on CT. The sections (a)–(d) are at levels (a)–(d) in Fig. 4.9. The sections should be regarded as being viewed from below **(i.e. the left of the thorax is on the right of the figure).** (a) *Section above the aortic arch*. Many large vessels and an anterior sausage shape are seen; the trachea has not bifurcated (black circle). Numerals refer to Fig. 4.9 and its legend. (b) *Section at the level of aortic arch*. A large oblique sausage shape representing the aortic arch is seen (ao); oes, oesophagus which is visible in all of the sections; svc, superior vena cava. (c) *Section below the aortic arch*. Both ascending (aao) and descending (dao) aortas are visible, the trachea is bifurcating and the pulmonary arteries are seen; pa, left pulmonary artery. (d) *Section at the level of pulmonary veins (pv)*. Lower lobe intrapulmonary arteries and bronchi are not shown in the diagram.

can provide a detailed image of emphysema (see Chapter 12) and interstitial lung disease. A 'ground glass' appearance on a high-resolution CT scan of a patient with idiopathic pulmonary fibrosis, for example, corresponds to a cellular pattern on histology whereas a 'reticular pattern' often indicates fibrosis with less active inflammation and less response to steroids (see Chapter 14). Modern CT scanners have the capacity to perform very rapid spiral images and this imaging technique combined with injection of radiocontrast material into a peripheral vein can be used to identify emboli in central pulmonary arteries in thromboembolic disease (see Chapter 16).

Positron emission tomography

Positron emission tomography (PET) scanning is being increasingly used in the diagnosis and staging of lung cancer. It is based on the concept that neoplastic cells have greater metabolic activity and a higher uptake of glucose than normal cells. ^{18}F-fluoro-2-deoxy-glucose (FDG) is a glucose analogue which is preferentially taken up by neoplastic cells after intravenous injection and which then emits positrons. PET scanning is particularly helpful in the differential diagnosis of an indeterminate **solitary pulmonary nodule**. Often such a nodule is small and not amenable to biopsy.

Calcification or lack of growth of the lesion over time suggest that the nodule is benign (e.g. hamartoma, healed tuberculous granuloma). If the patient is a smoker at high risk of cancer and otherwise fit it may be advisable to proceed directly to surgical resection of such a lesion without preoperative histological confirmation. Active accumulation of FDG in the lesion on PET scanning suggests malignancy. False-negative findings can occur in tumours <1 cm and false-positive uptake can occur in inflammatory conditions such as tuberculosis, sarcoidosis, histoplasmosis and coccidioidomycosis. PET scanning is also useful in the **staging of lung cancer** by detecting spread of the tumour to mediastinal lymph nodes.

Keypoints

- The chest X-ray has a key role in the investigation of lung disease. It should be studied in a systematic way and interpreted in the context of all clinical information.
- CT is more sensitive than the chest X-ray and is crucial in the staging of lung cancer, in assessing interstitial lung disease and in diagnosing pulmonary emboli.
- Ultrasonography is useful in assessing pleural effusions and may be used to guide placement of a chest drain in a loculated pleural effusion.
- PET is helpful in diagnosing and staging lung cancer.

Further reading

Hansell DM. Thoracic imaging. In: Gibson GJ, Geddes DM, Costabel U, Sterk PJ, Corrin B, eds. *Respiratory Medicine*. London: WB Saunders Co, 2003: 316–51.

Lynch DA, Godwin JD, Safrin S et al. High-resolution computed tomography in idiopathic pulmonary fibrosis. *Am J Respir Crit Care Med* 2005; **172**: 488–93.

Remy-Jardin M, Ghaye B, Remy J. Spiral computed tomography angiography of pulmonary embolism. *Eur Respir Monograph* 2004; **27**: 124–43.

Vansteenkiste JF. Imaging in lung cancer: position emission tomography scan. *Eur Respir J* 2002; **19** (Suppl. 35): 49–60.

Verschakelen JA, DeWever W, Bogaert J, Stroobants S. Imaging: staging of lung cancer. *Eur Respir Monograph* 2004; **30**: 214–44.

Part 3

Respiratory Diseases

Chapter 5

Upper respiratory tract infections and influenza

Introduction

Acute upper respiratory tract infections (URTIs) are a very common cause of morbidity, visits to doctors and absence from school or work. They are the most common respiratory complaint accounting for about **9% of all consultations in general practice**. A child suffers about eight, and an adult about four respiratory infections each year. Although unpleasant, most URTIs are mild and self-limiting, but a small number give rise to serious problems, most notably acute epiglottitis in children and influenza A in elderly patients debilitated by chronic underlying disease. Difficulties arise in distinguishing URTIs from more serious lower respiratory tract infections such as pneumonia (Fig. 5.1), and alertness combined with careful assessment and clinical judgement are required. Most URTIs are of viral origin but a variety of viruses and bacteria may produce the same clinical pattern of illness (e.g. pharyngitis, sinusitis).

Common cold

The common cold (coryza) is an acute illness characterised by rhinorrhoea, sneezing, nasal obstruction and sore throat (pharyngitis) with minimal fever or systemic symptoms. It may be caused by about 200 different strains of viruses including **rhinoviruses, coronaviruses, respiratory syncytial,** **parainfluenza** and **influenza viruses.** Infection is transmitted by droplet spread, and attack rates are highest in young children attending school who then transmit infection to their parents and siblings at home. The multiplicity of viral strains prevents the development of immunity. The bacterial flora of the nasopharynx remains unchanged for the first few days of the illness but then may show an increase in the number of *Haemophilus influenzae* and *Streptococcus pneumoniae* organisms, and there is the potential for secondary bacterial infection to occur with extension of infection beyond the nasopharynx, giving rise to sinusitis, otitis media, bronchitis or pneumonia. Most people with the common cold do not need to see their general practitioner and can be encouraged to manage the condition themselves or to seek advice from a pharmacist. No specific treatment is possible for the common cold but symptoms are often alleviated by use of paracetamol or aspirin.

Pharyngitis

Pharyngitis may occur as part of the common cold or as a separate illness. Most cases are caused by **viruses** (Table 5.1) but pharyngitis may also be caused by group A β-**haemolytic streptococci,** *Mycoplasma pneumoniae* or *Chlamydia pneumoniae*, for example. The patient complains of a sore throat and there is erythema of the pharynx often with enlargement of the tonsils. **Infectious**

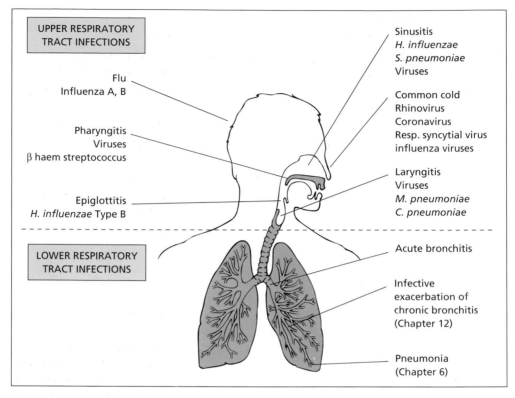

Figure 5.1 Acute respiratory infections.

mononucleosis (glandular fever) often involves pharyngitis but is also associated with lymphadenopathy and splenomegaly, and is caused by the Epstein–Barr (EB) virus. A blood film may show atypical mononuclear cells and the Monospot or heterophile antibody tests are positive. Characteristically, patients with infectious mononucleosis develop a rash if given amoxicillin as treatment of pharyngitis. It is not possible to distinguish between viral and bacterial pharyngitis on clinical grounds. β-haemolytic streptococci may be found on microbiology of a throat swab but this does not differentiate between active infection and a carriage state. Even when pharyngitis is caused by bacterial infection antibiotics are not usually necessary, as the illness tends to be self-limiting. Local extension of infection may result in otitis media, tonsillitis or quinsy (peritonsillar abscess). Streptococcal infection may be complicated by glomerulonephritis or rheumatic fever but these are rare nowadays.

Antibiotic treatment of pharyngitis is usually only given to severe or complicated cases. Streptococci are sensitive to penicillin V or amoxicillin. *Mycoplasma pneumoniae* or *Chlamydia pneumoniae* require a tetracycline or macrolide antibiotic (e.g. erythromycin, clarithromycin).

Sinusitis

Infection of the maxillary sinuses causes facial pain, nasal obstruction and discharge, often accompanied by fever and malaise. A variety of organisms may cause sinusitis including respiratory **viruses**, **Haemophilus influenzae**, **Streptococcus pneumoniae**, **Staphylococcus aureus** and **anaerobic bacteria**. In chronic sinusitis X-rays may show mucosal thickening, opacification or the presence of a fluid level in the sinus. Recurrent sinusitis may be accompanied by more widespread respiratory tract infection in patients with bronchiectasis caused

Table 5.1 Principal respiratory viruses.

Virus	Disease	Notes
Rhinovirus	Common cold, pharyngitis, chronic bronchitic exacerbations	More than 100 serotypes; identification and study difficult
Coronavirus	Common cold	Numerous serotypes; identification difficult
	Severe Acute Respiratory Syndrome (SARS)	SARS coronavirus (see Chapter 6)
Adenovirus	Pharyngitis, conjunctivitis, severe bronchitis in childhood, rarely severe pneumonia	About 30 serotypes
Respiratory syncytial virus	Bronchiolitis in infants, common cold in adults	One serotype, winter epidemics
Influenza A	Influenza—may be severe	Epidemics, continuous antigenic variation
Influenza B	Influenza	Milder illness, minor epidemics
Parainfluenza	Croup, other upper respiratory tract infections, some bronchiolitis	Serotypes 1–4, A and B
Measles	Measles, severe illness with pneumonia in immunocompromised	Vaccination effective
Cytomegalovirus	Silent infection or minor respiratory illness, pneumonia in immunosuppressed	One serotype
Herpes simplex	Stomatitis, rarely pharyngitis, pneumonia in immunosuppressed	One serotype, severe infection treatable with aciclovir or vidarabine
Herpes zoster	Pneumonia in adult infection	Severe infection treatable with aciclovir, leaves scattered calcific lesions
Coxsackie, enteroviruses and ECHO viruses	Minor part in respiratory infection, Coxsackie A may cause herpangina; B causes 'pleurodynia' and pericarditis/myocarditis	Local epidemics
EB virus	Pharyngitis, lymphadenitis, infectious mononucleosis	Heterophile antibody test, typical blood picture

by cystic fibrosis, hypogammaglobulinaemia or ciliary dyskinesia. Post-nasal drip from sinusitis is irritating to the larynx and is quite a common cause of a persistent cough. Sinusitis is usually treated with antibiotics (e.g. amoxicillin, trimethoprim), nasal decongestants (e.g. ephedrine) and analgesia (e.g. paracetamol). Surgical drainage may be necessary for relief of chronic sinusitis.

Acute laryngitis

This term is used when temporary hoarseness or loss of voice occurs with pharyngitis or the common cold, and is caused by oedema of the vocal cords. No treatment is necessary.

Croup

Croup (acute laryngotracheobronchitis) is usually caused by **viruses** such as parainfluenza virus, respiratory syncytial virus, influenza A and B, rhinoviruses, adenovirus and measles. Characteristically, the child develops a harsh barking cough with an upper respiratory infection and this may progress to stridor. Often no treatment is required but some children develop more severe lower respiratory infections and progressive respiratory distress requiring intubation and ventilation. Oral prednisolone is sometimes beneficial in severe croup and nebulised high-dose budesonide may be associated with more rapid recovery in less severely affected patients.

Acute epiglottitis

Epiglottitis is a very serious disease which is usually caused by virulent strains of *Haemophilus influenzae* type B, and there is often an accompanying septicaemia. Death may result from occlusion of the airway by the inflamed oedematous epiglottis. It is most common in children of about 2–3 years of age, but cases have also occurred in adults. The patient is ill with pyrexia, sore throat, laryngitis and painful dysphagia. Symptoms of upper airway obstruction may develop rapidly with stridor and respiratory distress. A lateral neck X-ray may show the epiglottic swelling. Blood cultures often isolate *Haemophilus influenzae* type B. Patients with suspected epiglottitis should be admitted to hospital and attempts at examining the upper airway should only be performed when facilities are available for tracheal intubation and ventilation. Because of possible amoxicillin resistance chloramphenicol or cefuroxime are appropriate antibiotics.

Influenza

Seasonal Influenza

Influenza is an acute illness characterised by pyrexia, malaise, myalgia, headache and prostration as well as upper respiratory symptoms. Lethargy and depression may persist for several days afterwards. Although the term 'flu' is used very loosely by the public, it is the systemic features which characterise true infection with the influenza viruses. Influenza virus type A undergoes frequent spontaneous changes in its haemagglutinin and neuraminidase surface antigens. Minor changes, referred to as '**antigenic drift**', result in outbreaks of seasonal influenza in the winter months each year. Major changes, referred to as '**antigenic shift**', result in epidemics and **pandemics** of infection reflecting the lack of immunity in the population to the new strain. Type B is more antigenically stable and produces less severe disease. Type C causes only mild sporadic cases of upper respiratory infection.

Influenza is highly infectious so that all members of a household often become ill together. Outbreaks of influenza cause considerable morbidity even in healthy adults. It is usually a self-limiting illness but can be complicated by bronchitis, otitis media and secondary bacterial pneumonia (e.g. *Staphylococcus aureus*, *Streptococcus pneumoniae* or *Haemophilus influenzae*). The greatest morbidity and mortality occur in patients who are elderly with underlying cardiac or respiratory disease and seasonal influenza outbreaks cause an average annual excess mortality of about 12 000 deaths in the UK.

The diagnosis of influenza can be confirmed by immunofluorescent microscopy of nasal secretions or by serology. **Oseltamivir** and **zanamivir** are drugs which reduce the replication of influenza viruses by inhibiting viral neuraminidase. Oseltamivir is given orally whereas zanamivir is only available by inhalation. These drugs have to be given within 48 hours of the onset of symptoms to be effective. They reduce the duration of illness by about 1 day and they may reduce complications in at-risk patients with severe influenza. They can also be given for post-exposure prophylaxis in at-risk adults not protected by vaccination. Vaccination remains the most effective way of preventing illness from seasonal influenza. However if new pandemic strains of influenza emerge it will take time to develop vaccines. **Amantadine** is an older antiviral agent which blocks the ion channel function of a protein in the influenza virus, but some strains are resistant to this drug and it is not currently recommended for the treatment of influenza in the UK. Use of aspirin or paracetamol relieves symptoms. Antibiotics are used when there are features of secondary bacterial infection (e.g. otitis media, sinusitis). Pneumonia associated with influenza may be severe and requires treatment with broad-spectrum antibiotics including flucloxacillin because of the risk of *Staphylococcus aureus* infection.

Influenza vaccination

The influenza vaccine is prepared each year using the virus strains most likely to be prevalent that year. The vaccine contains inactivated virus and is about 70–80% effective in protecting against infection. Where infection occurs despite vaccination it is usually less severe and associated with less morbidity and mortality than the disease seen in unvaccinated patients. Selective immunisation is recommended to protect those most at risk of serious illness or death from influenza. Annual vaccination is recommended for those with chronic respiratory disease (e.g. chronic obstructive pulmonary disease, asthma, bronchiectasis, etc.), chronic heart disease, renal failure, diabetes mellitus, immunosuppression and for elderly patients living in nursing homes.

Adverse reactions to influenza vaccine are usually mild, consisting of fever and malaise in some patients and local reactions at the site of injection. The vaccine is contraindicated in patients with egg allergy. Patients should be advised that the vaccine will not protect them from all respiratory viruses.

Pandemic influenza

Influenza pandemics have occurred sporadically and unpredictably over the last century. They arise when there are major changes in the haemagglutinin and neuraminidase surface antigens of the influenza A virus. In 1918 a pandemic of influenza caused by the H1N1 strain (Spanish flu) killed about 30 million people worldwide. There were further pandemics in 1957, caused by the H2N2 strain (Asian flu), and in 1968, caused by the H3N2 strain (Hong Kong flu), each killing about 1 million people worldwide. In recent years there is concern about the transmission of an avian strain of influenza (H5N1) from birds such as ducks and poultry to humans. This has occurred mainly in South East Asia and has produced severe influenza pneumonia in humans, with a high death rate. Spread of infection has been contained by slaughtering large numbers of birds in affected areas. There is the potential for such influenza viral strains to undergo mutations which might increase the capacity for transmission from human to human, which could then give rise to pandemic infection. During pandemics the number of patients with influenza can overwhelm the normal healthcare systems and contingency plans have been developed for such circumstances.

> ### Keypoints
>
> - Most upper respiratory infections are self-limiting, caused by viruses, and antibiotics are not usually indicated.
> - Seasonal influenza A causes an acute systemic illness with substantial morbidity and mortality, particularly in elderly at-risk patients.
> - Influenza A vaccine is prepared each year for the prevalent strains and gives effective protection against seasonal influenza.
> - Pandemic influenza occurs when there are major mutations in the virus which result in increased virulence and a lack of immunity in the population.

Further reading

British Infection Society, British Thoracic Society, Health Protection Agency in collaboration with the Department of Health. Pandemic flu: clinical management of patients with an influenza-like illness during an influenza pandemic. www.dh.gov.uk(search for 4615)

Husby S, Agertoft L, Mortensen S, Pedersen S. Treatment of croup with nebulised steroid (budesonide): a double-blind placebo controlled study. *Arch Dis Child* 1993; **68**: 352–6.

Little PS, Williamson I, Shvartzman P. Are antibiotics appropriate for sore throats? *BMJ* 1994; **309**: 1010–12.

Mansel JK, Rosenow EC, Smith TF, Martin JW. *Mycoplasma pneumoniae*. Chest 1989; **95**: 639–46.

Vernon DD, Sarnaik AP. Acute epiglottitis in children: a conservative approach to diagnosis and management. *Crit Care Med* 1986; **14**: 23–5.

Wilson R. Influenza vaccination. *Thorax* 1994; **49**: 1079–80.

Wong SSY, Yuen KY. Avian influenza virus infections in humans. *Chest* 2006; **129**: 156–68.

Chapter 6

Pneumonia

Lower respiratory tract infections

The lower respiratory tract, below the larynx, is normally sterile. Infections can reach the lungs by a number of routes: **inhalation, aspiration, direct inoculation** (e.g. stab wound to chest) and **blood borne** (e.g. from intravenous drug misuse). In some situations lower respiratory tract infection may be regarded as a *primary exogenous event* in which inhalation of a large dose of a virulent pathogen produces a severe infection in a previously healthy person. Thus, *Legionella pneumophila* may be inhaled from a contaminated water system, or *Chlamydia psittaci* from an infected bird resulting in a severe pneumonia. In other circumstances infection is a *secondary endogenous event.* Thus, a patient who is debilitated by major trauma and requiring endotracheal ventilation in an intensive therapy unit (ITU) may develop pneumonia. Typically in these circumstances the patient's oropharynx becomes colonised by Gram-negative enteric bacteria which are usually acquired from endogenous sources within the patient such as the upper gastrointestinal tract, subgingival dental plaque and periodontal crevices. These bacteria may then reach the lower airway by microaspiration.

Pneumonia

Pneumonia is a general term denoting inflammation of the gas exchange region of the lung.

Usually it implies **parenchymal lung inflammation caused by infection**, and the term 'pneumonitis' is sometimes used to denote inflammation caused by physical, chemical or allergic processes. Pneumonia is an important cause of morbidity and mortality in all age groups. Globally it is estimated that 5 million children under the age of 5 years die from pneumonia each year (95% in the developing countries). In the UK about 1 in 1000 of the population are admitted to hospital with pneumonia each year and the mortality in these patients is about 10%. There are about 3000 deaths from pneumonia each year in the age group 15–55 years. About 25% of all deaths in the elderly are related to pneumonia, although this is often the terminal illness in a patient with serious concomitant disease.

Classification in relation to clinical context (Fig. 6.1)

A microbiological approach to pneumonia focuses primarily on identification of the pathogen and its susceptibility to antibiotics. However, many of the major respiratory pathogens may be present in the oropharynx in a normal person so that identification of an organism in respiratory tract secretions may not be sufficient to implicate it as the cause of the illness. Conversely the same pathogen can cause various illnesses at different levels in the respiratory tract such as sinusitis, bronchitis or pneumonia, and different bacteria may cause an identical

Previously well infant
1 RSV
2 Adenovirus and other viruses
3 Bacterial

Previously ill infant
1 Staphylococcus
2 *E. coli* and Gram-negative bacteria
3 Viruses and opportunistic organisms

Children
1 Viruses
2 Pneumococcus
3 Mycoplasma
4 Others

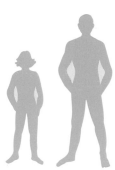

Previously fit adults
1 Pneumococcus
2 Mycoplasma
3 *H. influenzae*
4 Viruses
5 Staphylococcus
6 *Legionella*
7 Others

Previous respiratory illness;
elderly and debilitated
1 Pneumococcus
2 *H. influenzae*
3 Staphylococcus
4 *Klebsiella* and
   Gram-negative organisms

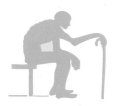

If no response think of:
TB, *Mycoplasma, Legionella,*
carcinoma

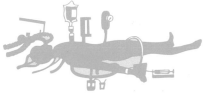

Severely immunocompromised
and AIDS (see Chapter 8):
1 Pneumocystis pneumonia
2 Cytomegalovirus
3 Adenovirus
4 Herpes simplex
5 Bacteria (*Legionella,*
   Staphylococcus, Pneumococcus)
6 Opportunistic mycobacteria;
   tuberculosis

Hospital-acquired pneumonia
1 Gram-negative bacteria
   (*Pseudomonas, Klebsiella,*
   Proteus)
2 Staphylococcus
3 Pneumococcus
4 Anaerobic bacteria, fungi
5 NB aspiration pneumonia
6 Others

Figure 6.1 Likely causes of pneumonia in different clinical circumstances. Age and previous health are important factors.

clinical syndrome such as pneumonia. A clinical approach to pneumonia focuses on the clinical context of the illness, the patient's previous health status and on the circumstances of the illness. Pneumonia is the result of a complex interaction between the **patient**, the **environment** and the **infecting organism**, and the pattern of the disease depends on the **virulence** of the pathogen and the **vulnerability** of the patient. The circumstances of the illness include the following:

● site of infection in the respiratory tract,
● age of the patient,

- community- or hospital-acquired infection,
- concurrent disease,
- environmental and geographical factors,
- severity of the illness and
- microbiology of the pneumonia.

Site of infection

The term 'chest infection' is an imprecise term often used by lay people to refer to non-specific respiratory symptoms. In assessing and treating respiratory tract infections it is important to define the site of infection as clearly as possible. **Upper respiratory tract infections** (above the larynx) are often viral in origin and self-limiting, not requiring treatment (see Chapter 5). **Lower respiratory tract infections** may affect the bronchial tree as **bronchitis**, or the lung parenchyma as **pneumonia**. Infective exacerbations of chronic bronchitis (see Chapter 12) are often caused by organisms of low virulence (e.g. non-typeable *Haemophilus influenzae*) when the patient's defences against infection are compromised by smoking-induced damage to the bronchial mucosa. Penetration of antibiotics into the scarred mucosa and viscid secretions may be difficult. Extension of bronchial infection into the surrounding lung parenchyma is often referred to as **bronchopneumonia**. Infection of the lung parenchyma with extensive consolidation of a lobe of a lung—**lobar pneumonia**—is usually caused by organisms of greater virulence (e.g. *Streptococcus pneumoniae*). Infection may spread to the pleura resulting in **empyema**, or to the bloodstream causing **septicaemia**.

Age of the patient

In **children** under the age of 2 years pneumonia is commonly caused by viruses such as respiratory syncytial virus (RSV), adenovirus, influenza and parainfluenza viruses. *Chlamydia trachomatis* infection may be transmitted to the infant from the mother's genital tract during birth resulting in pneumonia. In older children and **adults** of all ages *Streptococcus pneumoniae* is the most common cause of primary pneumonia. *Mycoplasma pneumoniae* infection is rare in the elderly and particularly

affects young adults. The incidence of pneumonia increases greatly in the **elderly** and the high frequency of underlying chronic diseases (e.g. chronic obstructive pulmonary disease (COPD), heart failure) in this group is associated with a high mortality.

Community- or hospital-acquired pneumonia

The characteristics of the patients and the spectrum of pathogens differ greatly depending on whether pneumonia is contracted in the community or in hospital. When pneumonia is acquired in the community it may be a primary infection in a previously healthy individual or it may occur in association with concomitant disease (e.g. COPD), but a few pathogens (notably *Streptococcus pneumoniae*) account for the majority of cases and Gram-negative organisms are rare. Most patients are treated at home with only about 25% needing hospital admission. The most important organisms identified as causing **community-acquired pneumonia** are as follows:

Streptococcus pneumoniae	50–60%
Mycoplasma pneumoniae	10%
Chlamydia pneumoniae	10%
Viruses (e.g. influenza)	10%
Haemophilus influenzae	5%
Staphylococcus aureus	3%
Legionella pneumophila	2%
Others	5%

Hospital-acquired (nosocomial pneumonia) is defined as pneumonia developing 2 or more days after admission to hospital for some other reason. It is therefore a secondary infection in patients with other illnesses. In these circumstances Gram-negative organisms (e.g. *Pseudomonas aeruginosa*, *Escherichia coli*) are the most important pathogens. A variety of factors, including use of broad-spectrum antibiotics and impaired host defences, promote the colonisation of the nasopharynx of hospitalised patients with Gram-negative organisms. Aspiration of infected nasopharyngeal secretions into the lower respiratory tract is facilitated by factors which compromise the defence mechanisms of the lung (e.g. endotracheal intubation in ITU) impaired cough associated with anaesthesia, surgery or cerebrovascular disease. The spectrum of causative organisms varies depending on the exact circumstances but the most common pathogens in **hospital-acquired pneumonia** are as follows:

Gram-negative bacteria	50%
Staphylococcus aureus	20%
Streptococcus pneumoniae	15%
Anaerobes and fungi	10%
Others (e.g. *Legionella pneumophila*)	5%

Concurrent disease

Alcohol misuse, malnutrition, diabetes and underlying **cardiorespiratory disease** predispose to pneumonia and are associated with a greatly increased mortality. Patients with **COPD** have impaired mucociliary clearance and organisms of quite low virulence (e.g. *Haemophilus influenzae*) may spread from the bronchi into the peribronchial lung parenchyma causing bronchopneumonia. Mortality from **influenza infection**, either as a cause of primary pneumonia or associated with secondary bacterial pneumonia, is highest in the **elderly**. **Aspiration pneumonia** is likely to occur in patients with impaired swallowing as a result of oesophageal or neuromuscular disease, or in patients with impaired consciousness (e.g. epileptic fits, anaesthesia).

Pneumonia in the immunocompromised (e.g. patients with human immunodeficiency virus (HIV) infection or receiving immunosuppressive drugs) is a very specific circumstance in which opportunistic infections (e.g. Pneumocystis pneumonia) are common. A particular approach to investigation and treatment is required in these circumstances (see Chapter 8). Patients who have undergone **splenectomy** are particularly vulnerable to pneumococcal pneumonia and septicaemia, and are usually given pneumococcal vaccination and maintained on lifelong penicillin prophylaxis.

Environmental and geographical factors

Although in some cases pneumonia arises by aspiration of endogenous infective organisms from the oropharynx, in other cases the patient's environment is the source of infection with the inhalation of infected droplets from **other patients** (e.g. influenza, tuberculosis), from an **animal source** (e.g. *Chlamydia psittaci* from birds, *Coxiella burnetti* from farm animals) or from other **environmental sources** (e.g. *Legionella pneumophila* from contaminated water systems).

Some infections have a particular **geographical distribution** (e.g. histoplasmosis in North America, typhoid in tropical countries) and need to be considered in patients who live in, or have recently visited, these areas. A knowledge of the **local pattern of prevalent infections** and **antibiotic resistance** in a community is important. For example, *Mycoplasma pneumoniae* infection particularly occurs in outbreaks about every 4 years and requires treatment with tetracycline or a macrolide (e.g. erythromycin) antibiotic. Although *Streptococcus pneumoniae* in the UK is usually sensitive to penicillin, about 30% of strains isolated in Spain are resistant and this should be borne in mind when choosing initial antibiotic therapy.

Severity of pneumonia (Fig 6.2)

Community-acquired pneumonia has a wide spectrum of severity from a mild self-limiting illness to a fatal disease. It is therefore vital to assess accurately the severity of the pneumonia, as this is an important factor in determining the choice of antibiotics, the extent of investigations and in deciding whether a patient should be treated **in hospital** rather than **at home** or in an **ITU** rather than on a general ward. Severe pneumonia can rapidly develop into multiorgan failure with respiratory, circulatory and renal failure. Patients who have certain core adverse prognostic features have a greatly increased risk of death: acute **confusion**, elevated **urea** (>7 mmol/L), increased **respiratory rate** (≥30/min) and low **blood pressure** (systolic <90 mmHg, diastolic <60 mmHg), age over 65 years. A **CURB-65 score** is useful in assessing the severity of pneumonia (Fig 6.2). Patients with severe pneumonia are likely to benefit from more intensive monitoring (arterial catheter, central venous catheter, urinary catheter) and treatment

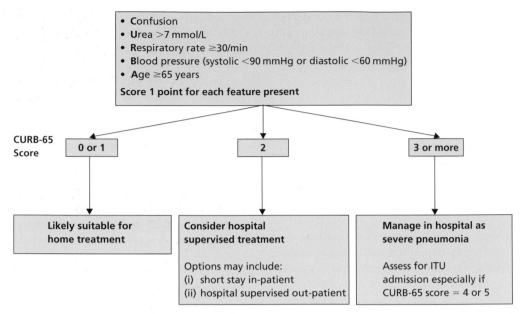

Figure 6.2 CURB-65 Severity Score. The severity of pneumonia can be assessed using a scoring system based on the key parameters of new onset confusion, an elevated urea, respiratory rate, blood pressure and age >65 years, giving a CURB-65 score. Patients with a score of >3 are at high risk of death and may need to be treated in an ITU. Patients with a score <1 may be suitable for treatment at home. (Reproduced with permission from the British Thoracic Society Guidelines for the management of community-acquired pneumonia—2004 update: www.brit-thoracic.org/guidelines).

(rapid correction of hypovolaemia, inotropic support, ventilatory support) in an ITU.

Clinical features

Patients with pneumonia typically present with **cough**, **purulent sputum** and **fever**, often accompanied by **pleuritic pain** and **dyspnoea**. There may be a history of a recent upper respiratory tract infection. Diagnosing the site and severity of respiratory tract infection is notoriously difficult and careful assessment combined with good clinical judgement is important. Early review of the situation is crucial in the event of deterioration because the severity of the illness is often underestimated by the patient and doctor alike. **Localised chest signs** such as crackles, dullness or bronchial breathing indicate pneumonia rather than bronchitis, for example, but may not always be present. Cyanosis and tachypnoea are features of respiratory failure. Rigors, high fever or prostration suggest septicaemia. Elderly patients, in particular, may

present with non-respiratory symptoms such as confusion.

The initial clinical approach focuses on an **assessment of the circumstances and severity** of the illness because these guide decisions as to how and where the patient should be treated. Rather than diagnosing a patient as having a 'chest infection' an effort should be made to use an appropriate descriptive phrase such as: 'a previously fit adult with severe community-acquired pneumonia and suspected septicaemia (rigors, prostration)' or 'probable bronchopneumonia (crackles) and respiratory failure (cyanosis) in a patient with COPD'.

Investigation

Patients with mild pneumonia which responds rapidly to antibiotics are usually treated at home and in this situation investigations do not usually influence management or outcome. Nonetheless, microbiology laboratories will often request that general practitioners send sputum and serology samples from some patients treated in the community so as to be able to alert clinicians to outbreaks of influenza or *Mycoplasma pneumoniae* for example, and to provide information on local patterns of bacterial resistance to antibiotics. More extensive investigations are indicated for patients requiring admission to hospital.

General investigations

- **Chest X-ray** (Fig. 6.3) confirms the diagnosis of pneumonia by demonstrating consolidation, detects complications such as lung abscess or empyema, and helps to exclude any underlying disease (e.g. bronchial carcinoma).
- **Haematology and biochemistry tests** are useful in assessing the severity of the disease.

Further investigations may be indicated if alternative diagnoses are being considered (e.g. computed tomographic angiography for pulmonary embolism). Where there is a suspicion of aspiration pneumonia a radiocontrast oesophagogram (e.g. 'Gastrografin swallow') is useful in assessing swallowing problems. Recurrent pneumonia may be an indication of an immunodeficiency state and tests such as measurement of immunoglobulin levels or HIV testing should be performed as appropriate. Measurement of C-reactive protein may help in differentiating pneumonia from non-infective diseases and in monitoring response to treatment.

Specific investigations

These are aimed at detecting the pathogen causing the pneumonia.

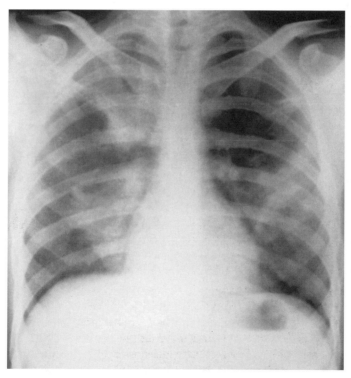

Figure 6.3 This 60-year-old man was admitted to hospital with a 2-week history of myalgia, headache, dyspnoea and cough without sputum. He was severely ill, cyanosed and confused with a fever of 39°C, tachycardia of 110/min, respiratory rate 40/min and blood pressure of 110/60 mmHg. Po_2 was 5.7 kPa (43 mmHg), Pco_2 4.9 kPa (37 mmHg), white cell count 4.6×10^9/L and urea 31 mmol/L. He had received amoxicillin for 6 days before admission without improvement. Chest X-ray shows extensive bilateral multilobar consolidation. He kept birds as a hobby and one of his budgerigars had died recently. The clinical diagnosis of psittacosis was subsequently confirmed by serology tests. He was treated with intravenous fluids, oxygen and tetracycline and recovered fully.

• **Sputum Gram stain** may give a valuable and rapid clue to the responsible organism in an ill patient.

• **Sputum culture** is the main test used to detect bacterial causes of pneumonia but contamination of the sample by oropharyngeal organisms, prior use of antibiotics and inability to produce sputum limit the sensitivity and specificity of the test.

• **Blood cultures** should be performed on all patients admitted to hospital but are positive in only about 15% of cases.

• **Pleural fluid** should be aspirated in all patients with pleural effusions and may yield a causative organism or reveal empyema (see Chapter 17).

• **Antigen detection tests** are available for some pathogens. Pneumococcal antigen may be identified in sputum, urine, pleural fluid or blood and may be positive in cases where prior antibiotics limit the sensitivity of cultures. Direct fluorescent antibody staining may detect *Legionella pneumophila* in bronchoalveolar lavage fluid, and tests for *Legionella* antigen in urine are available in some laboratories.

• **Serological tests** allow a retrospective diagnosis of the infecting organism if a rising titre is found between acute and convalescent samples. This is most useful for some viruses and pneumonia caused by atypical organisms such as *Mycoplasma pneumoniae* or *Chlamydia pneumoniae*.

Invasive investigations such as bronchoscopy with bronchoalveolar lavage may be indicated in severe pneumonia and in immunocompromised patients.

Treatment

General

Mild pneumonia in a fit patient can be treated **at home**. Admission to **hospital** is necessary for patients who demonstrate features of severe pneumonia, who have concomitant disease or who do not have adequate family help at home. The severity of the pneumonia should be formally assessed at the time of admission to hospital and elective transfer to an **ITU** should be considered for patients with severe disease.

Sufficient **oxygen** should be given to maintain arterial $P_{O_2} > 8$ kPa (60 mmHg) and oxygen saturation >90%. Adequate non-sedative **analgesia** (e.g. paracetamol or non-steroidal anti-inflammatory drugs) should be given to control pleuritic pain. **Fluid balance** should be optimised, using intravenous rehydration as required for dehydrated patients. Chest physiotherapy may be beneficial to patients with COPD and copious secretions but is not helpful in patients without underlying lung disease. Nutritional support (e.g. oral dietary supplements, nasogastric feeding) should be given in prolonged illnesses. The patient's general condition, pulse, blood pressure, temperature, respiratory rate and oxygen saturation should be monitored frequently and any deterioration should prompt reassessment of the need for transfer to ITU.

Antibiotic treatment

The initial choice of antibiotics is based upon an assessment of the circumstances and severity of the pneumonia. Treatment is then adjusted in accordance with the patient's response and the results of microbiology investigations. For **community-acquired pneumonia**, *Streptococcus pneumoniae* is the most likely pathogen and **amoxicillin** 500 mg–1 g t.d.s. orally is an appropriate antibiotic. Where there is a suspicion of an 'atypical pathogen' (e.g. *Mycoplasma pneumoniae*, *Chlamydia psittaci*) addition of a macrolide antibiotic, such as **erythromycin** 1 g q.d.s. or clarithromycin 500 mg b.d. is required. In **severe pneumonia** the initial antibiotic regimen must cover all likely pathogens and allow for potential antibiotic resistance, and intravenous **cefuroxime 1.5 g t.d.s. and clarithromycin 500 mg b.d.** are appropriate. In **hospital-acquired pneumonia**, Gram-negative bacteria are common pathogens, and a combination of an **aminoglycoside** (e.g. gentamicin) and a **third-generation cephalosporin** (e.g. ceftazidime) or an **anti-pseudomonal penicillin** (e.g. azlocillin) is commonly used.

Failure to respond or failure of the C-reactive protein level to fall by 50% within 4 days suggests the occurrence of a complication (e.g. empyema), infection with an unusual pathogen (e.g. *Legionella pneumophila*), the presence of antibiotic resistance or incorrect diagnosis (e.g. pulmonary embolism).

Specific pathogens

Pneumococcal pneumonia (Fig. 6.4)

Streptococcus pneumoniae is the causative organism in about **60% of community-acquired pneumonias** and in about 15% of hospital-acquired pneumonias. Research studies using tests for pneumococcal antigen suggest that it may account for many cases where no organism is identified. It is a Gram-positive coccus, which can cause infections at all levels in the respiratory tract including sinusitis, otitis media, bronchitis and pneumonia. Up to 60% of people carry *Streptococcus pneumoniae* as a **commensal in the nasopharynx** and infection is transmitted in airborne droplets. Nasopharyngeal carriage may progress to infection where there is a breach in the respiratory tract defences,

and smoking and viral infections are important factors disrupting surface defence mechanisms. There are many **different serotypes which vary in their virulence**, but virulent strains can render a previously fit and healthy person critically ill within a few hours. Pneumococcal infection in asplenic patients (e.g. post-splenectomy) is severe with a high mortality, such that these patients are usually given pneumococcal vaccination and long-term prophylactic phenoxymethylpenicillin 500 mg b.d. *Streptococcus pneumoniae* is usually **sensitive to penicillin antibiotics** (e.g. amoxicillin or benzyl penicillin) but antibiotic **resistance is an emerging problem** particularly in certain countries such as Spain, where about 30% of isolates are resistant, so that it is necessary to give broad antibiotic cover to a patient who has acquired pneumonia in a country with a high prevalence of antibiotic-resistant pneumococcus. **Pneumococcal vaccine** is recommended for patients with chronic lung disease, diabetes, renal and cardiac disease and for patients

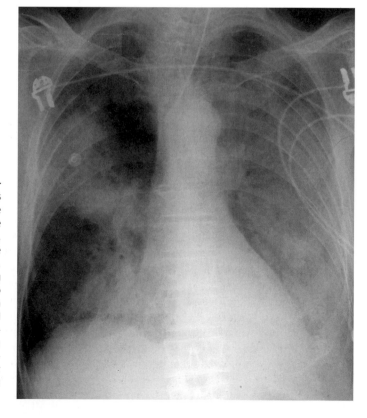

Figure 6.4 Pneumococcal pneumonia. This 70-year-old man was admitted to hospital with severe community-acquired pneumonia. He was confused with a fever of 39°C, respiratory rate 32/min, blood pressure 90/50 mmHg and a urea of 22 mmol/L. His CURB-65 score was 5, indicating severe pneumonia. He was admitted to the ITU but died despite treatment with antibiotics, mechanical ventilation and full supportive care. Blood cultures isolated *Streptococcus pneumonia.* In the UK about 1 in 1000 of the population are admitted to hospital each year with community-acquired pneumonia and about 10% of these patients die.

who are asplenic or immunodeficient (e.g. hypogam-maglobulinaemia, HIV).

Haemophilus influenzae pneumonia

Haemophilus influenzae is a **Gram-negative bacil-lus**. Virulent strains are encapsulated and divided into six serological types. ***Haemophilus influen-zae* type B (Hib)** is a virulent encapsulated form which causes **epiglottitis, bacteraemia, meningitis** and **pneumonia**. Hib vaccine is given to children to reduce the risk of meningitis and this vaccine also provides protection against epiglottitis. How-ever, it is the less virulent form of the organism—**non-typeable unencapsulated *Haemophilus influenzae*—**which is a common cause of respira-tory tract infection, predominantly where there has been damage to the bronchial mucosa by smoking or viral infection. *Haemophilus influenzae* often forms part of the normal pharyngeal flora. Deficient mucociliary clearance in patients with smoking-induced chronic bronchitis facilitates spread of the organism to the lower respiratory tract, where it gives rise to **exacerbations of COPD**. Spread of infection into the lung parenchyma causes **bronchopneumonia**. It is usually treated with **amoxicillin** but about 10% of strains are resistant and alternative antibiotics include co-amoxiclav (amoxicillin with clavulanic acid), trimethoprim and moxifloxacin.

Staphylococcal pneumonia

Staphylococcus aureus is a **Gram-positive coccus** which forms clusters resembling a bunch of grapes. Although it is a relatively uncommon cause of either community- or hospital-acquired pneumo-nia it may produce a very **severe illness with a high mortality**. It particularly occurs as a **sequel to influenza** so that anti-staphylococcal antibiotics should be given to patients who develop pneumo-nia after influenza. Infection may also reach the lungs via the bloodstream when staphylococcal bacteraemia arises from intravenous cannulae in hospitalised patients or from intravenous drug misuse, for example. The production of toxins may cause tissue necrosis with cavitation, pneumatocele formation and pneumothoraces. It is usually sen-sitive to cefuroxime but the standard treatment is with β-lactamase-resistant penicillins such as **flucloxacillin**.

Klebsiella pneumonia

Klebsiella pneumoniae is a **Gram-negative organism** which generally causes pneumonia only in **patients who have impaired resistance** to infection (e.g. **alcohol misuse, malnutrition, diabetes**) or under-**lying lung disease** (e.g. bronchiectasis). It often produces severe infection with destruction of lung tissue, **cavitation** and **abscess formation**. Treat-ment requires attention to the underlying disease state and prolonged antibiotic therapy, guided by the results of microbiology culture and sensi-tivity. Often a combination of a **third-generation cephalosporin** (e.g. ceftazidime) and an **amino-glycoside** (e.g. gentamicin) is appropriate.

Pseudomonas aeruginosa pneumonia

Pseudomonas aeruginosa is a **Gram-negative bacil-lus** which is a common cause of **pneumonia in hospitalised patients**, particularly those with neu-tropenia and those receiving endotracheal ventila-tion in ITU. It is usually treated with a combination of an aminoglycoside (e.g. gentamicin) and a third-generation cephalosporin (e.g. ceftazidime) or **anti-pseudomonal penicillin** (e.g. azlocillin).

Pneumonia caused by 'atypical pathogens'

'Atypical pathogens' is an imprecise term which is sometimes used in clinical practice to refer to certain pathogens which cause pneumonia such as *Mycoplasma pneumoniae*, chlamydial organisms and *Legionella pneumophila*. Characteristically, these organisms are **not sensitive to penicillins** and require treatment with **tetracycline or macrolide (e.g. erythromycin or clarithromycin)** antibiotics. These organisms are **difficult to culture** in the laboratory and the diagnosis is often made retro-spectively by demonstrating a rising antibody titre on serological tests.

Mycoplasma pneumonia

Mycoplasma pneumoniae is a small free-living organism, which does not have a rigid cell wall and which is therefore not susceptible to antibiotics such as penicillin which act on bacterial cell walls. Infection is transmitted from person to person by infected respiratory droplets. It **particularly affects children and young adults** although any age group may be affected. Infection typically occurs in **outbreaks every 4 years** and spreads throughout families, schools and colleges. *Mycoplasma pneumoniae* typically causes an initial upper respiratory tract infection with pharyngitis, sinusitis and otitis, followed by pneumonia in about 30% of cases. A variety of **extrapulmonary syndromes** may occur and may be related to immune responses to infection. These include lymphocytic meningoencephalitis, cerebellar ataxia, peripheral neuropathy, rashes, arthralgia, splenomegaly and hepatitis. **Cold agglutinins** to type O red cells are often present and haemolytic anaemia may occur. *Mycoplasma pneumoniae* causes significant protracted morbidity but is rarely life threatening.

Chlamydial respiratory infections

There are three chlamydial species which cause respiratory disease.

• *Chlamydia psittaci* is primarily an infection of **birds** which is transmitted to humans as a **zoonosis** (a disease contracted from animals) by inhalation of contaminated droplets. Psittacosis or ornithosis is the name given to the resultant illness which is often severe and characterised by high fever, headache, delirium, a macular rash and severe pneumonia.

• *Chlamydia pneumoniae* was identified as a respiratory pathogen in 1986. Infection is confined to **humans** and there is no avian or animal reservoir of infection. Infection with this organism is extremely common in all age groups and spreads directly from **person to person**, with **outbreaks occurring in families, schools and colleges**. It typically produces upper respiratory disease including pharyngitis, otitis and sinusitis but may also cause pneumonia which is usually mild.

• *Chlamydia trachomatis* is a common cause of sexually transmitted genital tract infection and **infants** may acquire respiratory tract infection with this organism from their mother's genital tract during birth.

Legionella pneumonia

Legionella pneumophila is a **Gram-negative bacillus** which is widely distributed in nature in **water**. The organism was first identified in 1976 when an outbreak of severe pneumonia affected delegates at a convention of the American Legion, who contracted infection from a contaminated humidifier system (**Legionnaires' disease**). In sporadic cases there is often no apparent source for the infection. Sometimes infection can be traced back to a **contaminated water system** such as a shower in a hotel room. Epidemics of infection may occur from a common source such as a contaminated humidification plant, water storage tanks or heating circuits. Infection does not spread from patient to patient. *Legionella pneumophila* typically causes a **severe pneumonia** with prostration, confusion, diarrhoea, abdominal pain and respiratory failure, with an associated high mortality. Direct fluorescent antibody staining may detect the organism in bronchoalveolar lavage fluid, and tests to detect *Legionella* antigen in urine are available, and allow rapid diagnosis. A combination of erythromycin and rifampicin is often used to treat severe *Legionella* pneumonia.

Severe acute respiratory syndrome

In 2003 there was a global epidemic of a severe acute respiratory syndrome (SARS) characterised by a severe pneumonia with a high mortality. The causative organism was identified as a new coronavirus which was named **SARS coronavirus**. The epidemic seems to have emerged from the Guandong province of China and then spread explosively with outbreaks in Hong Kong, Beijing, Taiwan, Singapore, Hanoi and Toronto. A particular feature of the epidemic was the very rapid global spread of infection by **airplane travel**.

For example, an infected person traveled by plane from Hong Kong to Toronto resulting in spread of infection to a new continent. Passengers on the plane and taxi drivers in contact with the index case developed infection. The SARS coronavirus is very virulent and highly infectious spreading from person to person by direct aerosol transmission or by indirect aerosolisation from contaminated surfaces. Secondary spread of infection from patients to **health care workers** and medical students was a major feature of the epidemic. Tertiary cases then occurred in the families of health care workers. Aerosolising procedures (e.g. nebulisation, suctioning of secretions, tracheal intubation) are particularly hazardous for transmission of infection from patients to health care workers. Many of the patients also had diarrhoea and in some outbreaks transmission may also have occurred by aerosolisation from sewage drainage systems. In total during 2003 approximately 8500 cases of SARS occurred in 29 countries with 916 deaths, giving a global case fatality of 11%. Patients presented with fevers, rigors, myalgia, cough, vomiting and diarrhoea and typically had peripheral consolidation on chest X-ray. Treatment mainly consisted of supportive care and 20% of patients required care on an ITU. Broad-spectrum antibiotics were given for potential secondary bacterial infections and some patients seemed to benefit from corticosteroids. Currently available anti-viral drugs do not seem to be effective against the SARS coronavirus. The global epidemic was brought to an end by late 2003 using **public health measures** including rapid case detection, case isolation, contact tracing and strict **infection control procedures** such as isolation of patients in negative pressure cubicles, use of respiratory protective masks, gowns, goggle and gloves. Vigilance is needed as there is the potential for the SARS coronavirus to re-emerge, and contingency plans emphasise the importance of infection control procedures in limiting spread of infection.

Keypoints

- Pneumonia is an important cause of morbidity and mortality in all age groups.
- About 1 in 1000 of the UK population are admitted to hospital each year with pneumonia and the mortality is 10%.
- *Streptococcus pneumoniae* is the most common cause of community-acquired pneumonia, but atypical pathogens (e.g. *Mycoplasma pneumoniae*) are also important such that treatment is often with a combination of amoxicillin and a macrolide antibiotic (e.g. clarithromycin).
- Gram-negative organisms (e.g. *Pseudomonas aeruginosa*) are the main cause of hospital-acquired pneumonia such that treatment is often with antibiotics such as ceftazidime, gentamicin or meropenem.
- The severity of community-acquired pneumonia should be assessed using the CURB-65 score (confusion, elevated urea, respiratory rate, blood pressure, age >65 years).

Further reading

American Thoracic Society. Guidelines for the management of adults with hospital-acquired, ventilation-associated and healthcare-associated pneumonia. *Am J Respir Crit Care Med* 2005; **171**: 388–416.

The British Thoracic Society guidelines for the management of community acquired pneumonia in adults 2004 update. www.brit-thoracic.org/guidelines

Hoare Z, Lim WS. Pneumonia: update on diagnosis and management. *BMJ* 2006; **332**: 1077–9.

Woodhead M, Blasi F, Ewig S et al. European Society Task Force. Guidelines for the management of adult lower respiratory tract infections. *Eur Respir J* 2005; **26**: 1138–80.

World Health Organization. Consensus document on the epidemiology of severe acute respiratory syndrome (SARS). http://www.who.int/csr/sars/guidelines/en/index.html

Chapter 7

Tuberculosis

Tuberculosis is an infection caused by *Mycobacterium tuberculosis* which may affect any part of the body but most commonly affects the lungs. It is spread by a person inhaling the bacterium in droplets coughed or sneezed out by someone with infectious tuberculosis.

Epidemiology

The World Health Organisation estimates that 2 **billion people (one-third of the world's population) have latent infection with *Mycobacterium tuberculosis*, 15–20 million people have active disease and 3 million deaths occur each year** from tuberculosis (95% in the developing world). One hundred years ago in the UK more than 30 000 people died from tuberculosis each year (about the same as for lung cancer at present). Mortality and notification rates declined steadily from 1900 onwards because of improvement in nutritional and social factors, with a sharper decline occurring from the late 1940s onwards after the introduction of effective treatment (Fig. 7.1). Notification rates in England and Wales reached a low point of about 5000 a year in 1987 but have increased again to about 6500 a year recently. This increased incidence of tuberculosis is mainly seen in inner city areas, particularly London, and the risk is highest in ethnic minority groups. The notification rates for tuberculosis are highest in the Black African (211 per 100 000 population), Pakistani (145 per 100 000) and Indian (104 per

100 000) ethnic groups and lowest in the white ethnic group (4 per 100 000). The recent increase in notification rates is partly due to patterns of immigration and increasing international travel. Other groups of people with a high incidence of tuberculosis are the homeless, those misusing drugs and alcohol and people co-infected with the human immunodeficiency virus (HIV). In younger age groups tuberculosis is often newly acquired infection whereas in the older age groups it is often reactivation of latent infection acquired many years previously. Factors which reduce resistance and precipitate reactivation include ageing, alcohol misuse, poor nutrition, debility from other diseases, use of immunosuppressive drug therapy and co-infection with HIV. In the UK, overlap between the population with HIV infection (mainly young white men) and the population with tuberculosis (mainly older white people and younger immigrants from the Indian subcontinent) is limited so that only 5% of patients with acquired immune deficiency syndrome (AIDS) have tuberculosis and about 3% of patients with tuberculosis are identified as having HIV infection. However, **4.5 million people worldwide are estimated to be co-infected with HIV and tuberculosis** (98% in developing countries).

Clinical course (Fig. 7.2)

The clinical course of tuberculosis often evolves over many years and represents a complex interaction

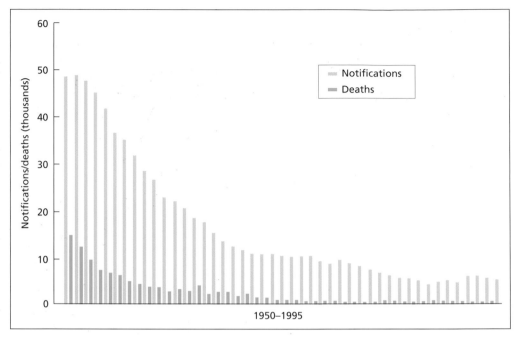

Figure 7.1 Notifications of tuberculosis and deaths in England and Wales, 1950–1995. Notifications of tuberculosis have declined from about 50 000 in 1950 to 5000 in 1987, since when notifications have increased to about 6500 per year. The recent increase is related to factors such as immigration, international travel and co-infection with HIV. (Reproduced with permission from *The Prevention and Control of Tuberculosis in the United Kingdom*, Department of Health, 1996.)

between the infecting organism (*Mycobacterium tuberculosis*) and the person's specific immune response and non-specific resistance to infection. Traditional descriptions of tuberculosis divide the disease into two main patterns, **primary** and **post-primary** tuberculosis, although these are mainly based upon the characteristic evolution of the disease in the days before effective chemotherapy.

Primary tuberculosis

Primary tuberculosis is the pattern of disease seen with **first infection** in a person (often a child) **without specific immunity** to tuberculosis. Infection is acquired by inhalation of organisms from an infected individual, and the initial lesion typically develops in the peripheral subpleural region of the lung followed by a reaction in the hilar lymph nodes. The **primary complex** appears on chest X-ray as a peripheral area of consolidation (Gohn focus) and hilar adenopathy. Occasionally,

erythema nodosum develops at this stage. An immune response develops, the tuberculin test becomes positive and **healing** often takes place. This stage of the disease is often asymptomatic but may leave calcified nodules on chest X-rays representing the healed primary focus. Active **progression** of first infection may occur. Bronchial spread of infection may cause progressive consolidation and cavitation of the lung parenchyma, and pleural effusions may develop. Lymphatic spread of infection may cause progressive lymph node enlargement, which in children may compress bronchi with obstruction, distal consolidation and the development of collapse and bronchiectasis. Bronchiectasis of the middle lobe is a very typical outcome of hilar node involvement by tuberculosis in childhood. Haematogenous spread of infection results in early generalisation of disease which may cause miliary tuberculosis, and the lethal complication of tuberculous meningitis (particularly in young children). Infection spread during

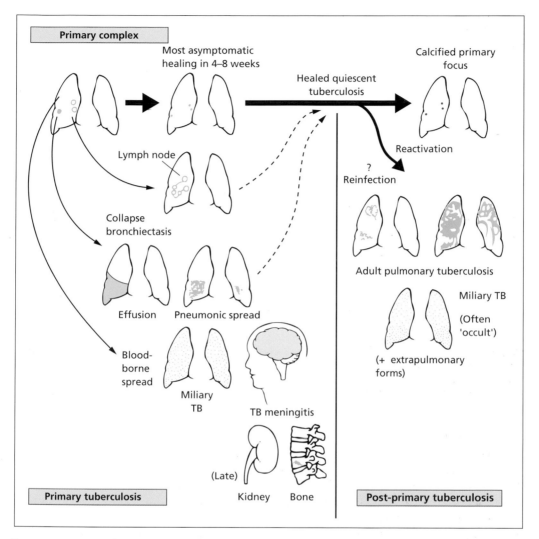

Figure 7.2 Summary of the natural history of tuberculosis.

this initial illness may lie **dormant** in any organ of the body (e.g. bone, kidneys) for many years only to **reactivate** many years later.

Post-primary tuberculosis

Post-primary tuberculosis is the **pattern of disease seen after the development of specific immunity**. It may occur following direct progression of the initial infection or result from endogenous **reactivation** of infection or from exogenous **re-infection** (inhalation of *Mycobacterium tuberculosis* from another infected individual) in a patient who has had previous contact with the organism and has developed a degree of specific immunity. Reactivation particularly occurs in old age and in circumstances where immunocompetence is impaired (e.g. illness, alcohol misuse, immunosuppressive drug treatment). The lungs are the most usual site of post-primary disease and the apices of the lungs are the most common pulmonary site.

Diagnosis

Clinical features

Definitive diagnosis requires identification of *Mycobacterium tuberculosis* because the clinical features of the disease are non-specific. The most typical **chest symptoms** are persistent cough, sputum production and haemoptysis. **Systemic symptoms** include fever, night sweats, anorexia and weight loss. A range of **chest X-ray** abnormalities occur (Figs 7.3 and 7.4). Cavitating apical lesions are characteristic of tuberculosis but such lesions may also be caused by lung cancer. Irregular mottled shadowing (particularly of the lung apices), streaky fibrosis, calcified granuloma, miliary mottling, pleural effusions and hilar gland enlargement may all be features of tuberculosis.

Diagnosis depends on the doctor having a high level of awareness of the many presentations of tuberculosis and undertaking appropriate investigations (e.g. sputum **acid- and alcohol-fast bacilli** (AAFB) staining and culture for tuberculosis) in patients with persistent chest symptoms or abnormal X-rays. A high index of suspicion is required in assessing patients who have recently immigrated from a high-prevalence area (e.g. Africa, Indian subcontinent), and in patients at risk for reactivation of infection because of factors which lower their resistance (age, alcohol misuse, debilitating disease, use of immunosuppressive drugs).

Although tuberculosis most commonly affects the lungs, **any organ in the body may be involved** and the diagnosis needs to be considered in patients with a **pyrexia of unknown origin** and in patients

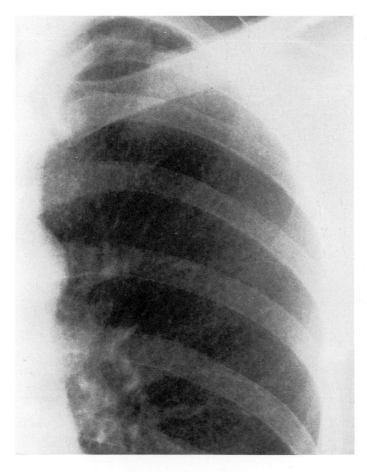

Figure 7.3 This 24-year-old man presented with malaise, fever and weight loss without any respiratory symptoms. Six months previously he had immigrated to the UK from Pakistan. X-ray shows multiple 1–2 mm nodules throughout both lungs characteristic of miliary tuberculosis. Sputum and bronchoalveolar lavage did not show acid- and alcohol-fast bacilli (AAFB). Transbronchial biopsies, however, showed caseating granulomas characteristic of tuberculosis. His symptoms resolved and the chest X-ray appearances returned to normal after 6 months of anti-tuberculosis chemotherapy.

with a variety of indolent chronic lesions (e.g. in bone, kidney or lymph nodes). The term **miliary tuberculosis** refers to a situation where there has been widespread haematogenous dissemination of tuberculosis, usually with multiple 'millet-seed' size nodules evident on chest X-ray. Chest symptoms are often minimal and typically the patient is ill and pyrexial with anaemia and weight loss.

Laboratory diagnosis

Identification of *Mycobacterium tuberculosis* by laboratory tests may take some time and anti-tuberculosis treatment may have to be commenced based on clinical and radiological features while awaiting the results of laboratory tests. Once the diagnosis is suspected, repeated **sputum** samples should be examined by the **Ziehl–Neelsen** (ZN) method

looking for AAFB which appear as red rods on a blue background. **Sputum cultures** require special media (e.g. Löwenstein–Jensen medium) and the tubercle bacillus grows slowly taking 4–7 weeks to give a positive culture and a further 3 weeks for the in vitro testing of antibiotic sensitivity. **Biopsy** of an affected site (e.g. pleura, lymph node, liver, bone marrow) may show the characteristic features of **caseating granuloma** (central cheesy necrosis of a lesion formed by macrophages, lymphocytes and epithelial cells). Biopsy specimens should also be submitted for mycobacterial cultures. Newer techniques are being developed to improve the speed, sensitivity and specificity of the laboratory diagnosis of tuberculosis. The **Bactec radiometric system**, for example, uses a liquid medium containing a radioactively labelled ^{14}C-labelled substance which releases $^{14}CO_2$ when metabolised,

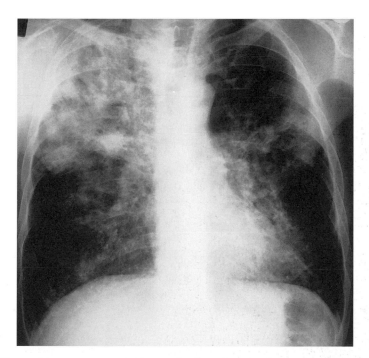

Figure 7.4 This 68-year-old man was persuaded to consult a doctor because of a 6-month history of cough, haemoptysis, night sweats and weight loss. He suffered from alcoholism and lived in a hostel for homeless men. His chest X-ray shows cavitating consolidation throughout the right upper lobe with further areas of consolidation in the left upper and right lower lobes. Sputum acid- and alcohol-fast bacilli (AAFB) stains were positive and cultures yielded *Mycobacterium tuberculosis* sensitive to standard drugs. He was treated with directly observed anti-tuberculosis therapy. Six of 38 residents of the hostel were found to have active tuberculosis. DNA fingerprinting techniques showed that this cluster of six cases was caused by three different strains of *Mycobacterium tuberculosis* arising as a result of both reactivation of latent tuberculosis in debilitated elderly men and spread of infection within the hostel.

and detection of this reflects the growth of *Mycobacterium tuberculosis*. DNA techniques using the **polymerase chain reaction** are being developed and may, for example, prove useful in detecting evidence of infection in cerebrospinal fluid in tuberculous meningitis. **DNA fingerprint techniques make it possible to distinguish different strains of *Mycobacterium tuberculosis*.** This can give useful insights into the likely sources and spread of infection and help assess the relative contribution of newly acquired and reactivated infection in different populations.

Treatment (Table 7.1)

Before effective antibiotics became available in the late 1940s, about 50% of patients with sputum-positive tuberculosis died of the disease. Patients were admitted to sanatoria for bed rest, 'sunshine and fresh air' therapy and nutritional support in an attempt to enhance their own resistance to the disease. When large tuberculous cavities developed in the lungs attempts were made to collapse the cavities by inducing an artificial pneumothorax, crushing the phrenic nerve, instilling various materials outside the pleura to compress the lung (plombage) or performing thoracoplasty, whereby the ribs were excised and the lung compressed against the mediastinum (Fig. 7.5). In the late 1940s **streptomycin** and **para-amino salicylic acid** (PAS) were introduced into clinical practice and the outlook for patients with tuberculosis was revolutionised. It soon became apparent that treatment had to be **prolonged** and **combinations** of antibiotics had to be used because of the capacity of the tubercle bacillus to lie dormant in lesions for long periods and to develop resistance to antibiotics.

The current standard treatment of tuberculosis consists of **6 months** of **rifampicin** and **isoniazid,**

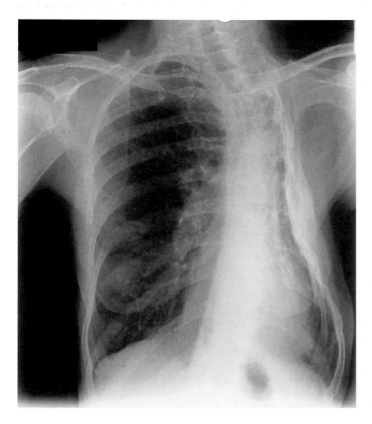

Figure 7.5 Thoracoplasty. Before effective antibiotics became available in the late 1940s about 50% of patients with sputum-positive tuberculosis died of the disease. At that time attempts were sometimes made to collapse large tuberculous cavities by performing a thoracoplasty, an operation in which the ribs were resected and the lung was compressed against the mediastinum.

supplemented by **pyrazinamide and ethambutol** for the first 2 months. All drugs are usually given in a single daily dose. Rifampicin and isoniazid are bactericidal drugs which kill extracellular bacilli which are actively metabolising. Both rifampicin and pyrazinamide are effective against intracellular bacilli, within macrophages. Prolonged treatment is needed to eradicate bacilli lying dormant. The use of the combination of drugs also prevents the emergence of resistance from the small number of bacilli which are naturally resistant to any one of the antibiotics. Ethambutol is bacteriostatic and is included in the treatment regimen to prevent the emergence of resistance to other drugs. It may be omitted in patients with a low risk of resistance to isoniazid (i.e. white patients who have not had previous anti-tuberculosis treatment and who do not have HIV infection). Patients from ethnic minority groups have a significantly higher risk of resistance to isoniazid and other drugs, and should be commenced on the four-drug combination. Meticulous **supervision** of treatment is essential and patients should be seen at least monthly for prescription of medication, checking of **compliance** with treatment and monitoring for side-effects (e.g. liver function tests). Errors in the prescription of medication or failure of the patient to comply with treatment may have serious consequences with the emergence of resistant organisms. **Directly observed therapy** should be instituted for patients who have difficulty complying with treatment, whereby the patient is observed to ensure that he or she swallows the medication. Sometimes this can be achieved by giving high doses of the anti-tuberculosis medication three times per week with the patient attending a hospital or general practice clinic to be given the medication under the supervision of a doctor or nurse. Flexible strategies are required to ensure compliance of patients with social (e.g. homelessness) or psychological (e.g. alcohol misuse, mental illness) problems and there is an important role for community health workers or trained laypersons in these circumstances.

At present, **drug-resistant tuberculosis** is rare in the initial treatment of patients from the white ethnic group in the UK, but is more common in patients who have had previous treatment or who come from Africa or the Indian subcontinent. Overall about 7.8% of isolates of *Mycobacterium tuberculosis* are resistant to isoniazid, 1.7% are resistant to rifampicin and 1.2% have multiple drug resistance. **Multidrug-resistant tuberculosis** results from inadequate previous treatment. The development of resistant organisms in a patient failing to comply with treatment may make the tuberculosis very difficult to treat, and such a patient poses a risk to public health because he or she may infect others with drug-resistant tuberculosis. Some outbreaks of multidrug-resistant tuberculosis have occurred in prisons and hospitals with high mortality rates.

Table 7.1 Treatment of tuberculosis.

Drug	Dose Children	Adult	Duration	Adverse effects
Isoniazid	10 mg/kg	300 mg	6 months	Hepatitis, neuropathy
Rifampicin	10 mg/kg	<50 kg 450 mg	6 months	Hepatitis, rashes
		≥50 kg 600 mg		Enzyme induction
Pyrazinamide	35 mg/kg	<50 kg 1.5 g	Initial	Hepatitis, rashes
		≥50 kg 2.0 g	2 months	Elevated uric acid
Ethambutol	15 mg/kg	15 mg/kg	2 months	Optic neuritis

- 6 months of rifampicin and isoniazid, with pyrazinamide and ethambutol for first 2 months
- Monitor treatment meticulously (e.g. monthly review)
- Check compliance
- Use directly observed therapy if problems with compliance
- Notify the diagnosis to Public Health Authorities
- Contact tracing of close family contacts.

The most dangerous of the **adverse reactions** to anti-tuberculosis treatment is **hepatotoxicity**, and patients should be advised to stop treatment and report for medical advice if they develop fever, vomiting, malaise or jaundice. Isoniazid, rifampicin and pyrazinamide may all cause hepatitis and allergic reactions such as **rashes**. Isoniazid may cause a **peripheral neuropathy** and this is preventable by pyridoxine 10 mg/day, which is given routinely to those at risk of neuropathy (e.g. patients with diabetes or alcohol misuse). Intermittent rifampicin may cause 'flu-like' symptoms, and the **induction of microsomal hepatic enzymes** reduces the serum half-life of drugs such as warfarin, steroids, phenytoin and oestrogen contraceptives so that patients may need adjustment in dosage of medications and may need to use alternative contraceptive measures. Rifampicin produces a reddish discoloration of urine (which may be used to monitor compliance) and may cause staining of soft contact lenses. Pyrazinamide sometimes causes initial facial flushing, and may cause an **elevation of uric acid levels** with arthralgia. Ethambutol causes a dose-related **optic neuropathy**, which is rare at doses below 15 mg/kg/day. Patients should have their visual acuity checked before starting treatment and should be warned to stop the drug if visual symptoms occur, and the drug should be avoided if possible in patients with impaired renal function or pre-existing visual problems.

Latent tuberculosis

The term **'latent tuberculosis'** refers to the situation where a person has been infected with *Mycobacterium tuberculosis* at some time but does not currently have active disease. The immune response has controlled the primary infection but all viable organisms might not have been eliminated. It is estimated that there is a 5–10% risk of a person with latent tuberculosis developing active disease at some stage over the course of their life. The greatest risk of progression to disease is within 2 years of the initial infection and this is particularly relevant when undertaking contact tracing procedures of people who may have acquired infection recently from a patient with active tuberculosis. Factors which increase the risk of reactivation of latent infection include ageing, alcohol misuse, poor nutrition, co-infection with HIV and use of immunosuppressive drugs. Recently, for example, tumour necrosis factor alpha antagonists are being used in the treatment of Crohn's disease and rheumatoid arthritis, and these immunosuppressive treatments are associated with a significant risk of reactivation of latent tuberculous infection such that latent infection should be sought and treated before starting such treatments. People with latent tuberculosis are asymptomatic and usually have a normal chest X-ray. Detection of latent infection depends on demonstrating an immune response to *Mycobacterium tuberculosis* using a tuberculin test or an interferon-gamma-based blood test.

Tuberculin testing (Fig. 7.6)

Hypersensitivity to the tubercle bacillus can be detected by the intradermal injection of a purified protein derivative (PPD) of the organism. The response is of the type IV cell-mediated variety and results in a raised area of induration and reddening of the skin. In the **Mantoux test** 0.1 mL of tuberculin solution is injected intradermally (not subcutaneously) and the test is read at 48–72 hours. A positive result is indicated by redness and induration at least 10 mm in diameter. If active tuberculosis is suspected the lowest dilution may be used initially to prevent a severe reaction, and higher concentrations used if there is no reaction. The **Heaf test** is performed with a spring-loaded needled 'gun'. A drop of undiluted PPD (100 000 TU/mL) is placed on the volar surface of the forearm and the 'gun' is used to puncture through the PPD solution. The reaction is graded from I to IV according to the formation of papules and the extent of induration. A positive tuberculin test indicates the presence of hypersensitivity to tuberculin resulting from either previous infection with tubercle bacillus or from bacillus Calmette–Guérin (BCG) vaccination. A weak reaction may be non-specific and indicate contact with other non-tuberculous environmental mycobacteria. A strongly positive test in a child who has

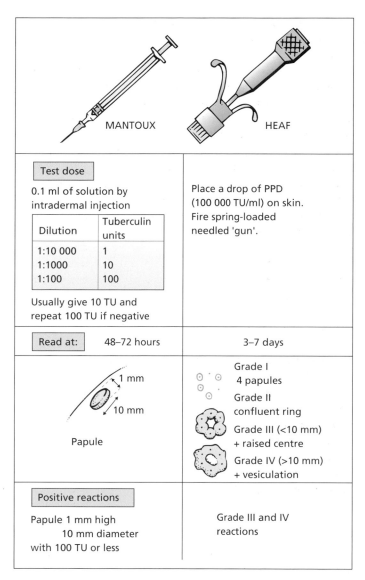

Figure 7.6 Tuberculin testing. In order to standardise procedures the Mantoux test is nowadays preferred to the previous Heaf test.

not received BCG vaccination is likely to indicate primary infection. If there is evidence of active disease, full anti-tuberculosis treatment is required; if there is no evidence of active disease chemoprophylaxis is advisable. A source amongst adult contacts of the child must be carefully sought. A negative tuberculin test makes active tuberculosis unlikely and indicates a lack of immunity so that BCG vaccination is recommended.

Interferon-gamma blood tests

Tuberculin skin tests lack specificity in diagnosing *Mycobacterium tuberculosis* infection since a positive reaction may be due to previous BCG vaccination or to exposure to non-tuberculous mycobacteria. In recent years laboratory assays have been developed which measure the release of interferon gamma from a patient's T-cells when exposed to specific antigens from *Mycobacterium tuberculosis*.

There are currently two such assays available in the UK: the Quantiferon Gold assay (Cellestis Limited, Australia) and the T-spot TB assay (Oxford Immunotec, Oxford, UK). These tests require only a single blood test but it needs to be analysed in the laboratory within a few hours. These interferon-gamma blood tests are likely to be most useful in more specific diagnosis of latent *Mycobacterium tuberculosis* infection.

Control

Treating active disease

Prompt **identification** and **treatment** of patients with active tuberculosis limits the spread of infection. Sputum-positive patients (AAFB positive) should be considered as potentially infectious until they have completed 2 weeks of treatment. The patient's family will already have been exposed to the risk of infection so that segregation of the patient from contact with his or her family at the time of diagnosis is not useful, and most patients can be treated as outpatients. Where patients with suspected or confirmed tuberculosis are admitted to hospital they should be kept in a single room. Particular care is required if the patient has multidrug-resistant tuberculosis and these patients should be treated in a negative pressure ventilation room to prevent transmission of infection to other patients or health-care workers.

Contact tracing

When a diagnosis of tuberculosis is made there is a statutory requirement in the UK for the doctor to **notify** the patient to the public health authorities who are then responsible for undertaking **screening of contacts**. The index patient may have acquired infection from, or transmitted infection to, someone in his or her close environment. It is usual to limit contact tracing to household contacts and to close friends sharing a similar level of contact with the index patient. If initial investigations reveal a large number of contacts with tuberculosis, consideration should be given to widening the circle of contacts who are offered screening. Typically about 1–3% of close contacts of smear-positive cases are found to have active disease, and many more have latent infection.

Screening of contacts consists of a combination of checking for symptoms of tuberculosis, **chest X-ray**, **tuberculin testing**, **interferon-gamma tests** and assessment of **BCG status**. Most cases of active tuberculosis are found at the first clinic visit in unvaccinated close contacts of smear-positive disease. If the contact has not had **BCG vaccination** a tuberculin test is performed and if this is negative vaccination is recommended. For children a tuberculin test is the usual initial screening test. Children with a strongly positive tuberculin test should have a chest X-ray. A strongly positive tuberculin test with a normal chest X-ray suggests that the child has been infected with tubercle bacillus has not developed active disease but remains at risk of doing so in the future. The risk of future activation of such latent infection is reduced by **chemoprophylaxis** which consists of treatment for 6 months with isoniazid alone, or for 3 months with isoniazid and rifampicin. In latent tuberculosis there are many thousand times fewer bacteria than in active tuberculosis and treatment with a single drug for 6 months or two drugs for 3 months is sufficient to kill dormant bacteria. Those with a negative tuberculin test should have it repeated 6 weeks later (to ensure they are not in the process of developing immunity to recently acquired infection), and if they remain tuberculin-negative BCG vaccination is advisable.

Screening of immigrants

Immigrants from areas with a high prevalence of tuberculosis (e.g. Africa, Indian subcontinent) should be screened for tuberculosis on arrival in a country of low prevalence such as the UK. Adults should have a chest X-ray and children should have a tuberculin test. Thereafter the procedure is as for close contacts, with treatment of active disease, chemoprophylaxis of latent infection or BCG vaccination as appropriate.

BCG vaccination

BCG is a live attenuated strain of tuberculosis which **provides about 75% protection against tuberculosis for about 15 years**. It is given by intradermal injection (not subcutaneous injection) and produces a local skin reaction. In the UK BCG vaccination used to be offered to children at the age of 13 years. This policy has now been changed from routine to **targeted vaccination** whereby BCG vaccination is offered to infants in communities with a high incidence of tuberculosis (>40 per 100 000) and to unvaccinated individuals who come from, or whose parents come from, countries with a high prevalence of tuberculosis.

Non-tuberculous mycobacteria (atypical opportunist mycobacteria)

There are a number of other mycobacteria that can cause pulmonary disease and that do not belong to the *Mycobacterium tuberculosis* complex. These are called 'atypical' or 'opportunist' mycobacteria and the most common of these are **Mycobacterium kansasii, Mycobacterium avium-intracellulare** complex, **Mycobacterium malmoense** and **Mycobacterium xenopi**. They are widespread in nature and can be found in water and soil so that sometimes contamination of clinical specimens occurs from environmental sources. They act as low-grade pathogens which do not usually pose a risk to normal individuals. Infections occur mainly in patients with impaired immunity (e.g. AIDS, see Chapter 8) or in those with damaged lungs (e.g. advanced emphysema or lung cavities from previous *Mycobacterium tuberculosis* infection). They are often associated with chronic symptoms such as cough, sputum production, haemoptysis and weight loss. Diagnosis is made on the basis of their characteristics on laboratory culture tests. Treatment is often difficult requiring prolonged (e.g. 2 years) treatment with rifampicin and ethambutol because these organisms often show resistance to some standard anti-tuberculosis antibiotics. Some more recently developed antibiotics (e.g. clarithromycin

or ciprofloxacin) may be useful in treatment. These organisms are low-grade pathogens and do not pose a threat to contacts of infected patients so that there is no need for contact tracing procedures.

Keypoints

- Worldwide, 2 billion people have latent infection with *Mycobacterium tuberculosis* and 15–20 million people have active tuberculosis.
- In the UK the incidence of tuberculosis is highest in the African, Pakistani and Indian ethnic groups, in homeless people and in people with reduced immunity because of ageing, alcohol misuse, poor nutrition, immunosuppressive drug treatments and co-infection with HIV.
- Diagnosis depends on having a high level of awareness of the presentations of tuberculosis and undertaking appropriate investigations (e.g. sputum AAFB staining) to identify *Mycobacterium tuberculosis*.
- Treatment consists of 6 months of rifampicin and isoniazid with pyrazinamide and ethambutol for the first 2 months.
- Control of tuberculosis involves detection and meticulous treatment of cases of active tuberculosis, notification of the diagnosis to the public health authorities, contact tracing to detect active or latent infection in contacts of the index case, and targeted vaccination of groups with a high incidence of tuberculosis.

Further reading

American Thoracic Society/Centers for Disease Control and Prevention/Infectious Diseases Society of America: Controlling tuberculosis in the United States. *Am J Respir Crit Care Med* 2005; **172**: 1169–227.

British Thoracic Society. Chemotherapy and management of tuberculosis in the United Kingdom. *Thorax* 1998; **53**: 536–48.

British Thoracic Society. Management of opportunist mycobacterial infections: Joint Tuberculosis Committee guidelines. *Thorax* 2000; **55**: 210–18.

British Thoracic Society. Recommendations for assessing risk and for managing *Mycobacterium tuberculosis* infection and disease in patients due to start anti-TNF-*á* treatment. *Thorax* 2005; **60**: 800–5.

Davies PDO, Drobniewski F. The use of interferon-gamma-based blood tests for the detection of latent tuberculosis infection. *Eur Respir J* 2006; **28**: 1–3.

Fine P. Stopping routine vaccination for tuberculosis in schools. *BMJ* 2005; **331**: 647–8.

National Institute for Health and Clinical Excellence. Clinical Guideline 33: Tuberculosis: clinical diagnosis and management of tuberculosis, and measures for its prevention and control. London, NICE, 2006. www.nice.org.uk

Chapter 8

Respiratory disease in HIV and immunocompromised patients

Acquired immune deficiency syndrome

Acquired immune deficiency syndrome (AIDS) was first recognised in 1981 when clusters of cases of Kaposi's sarcoma and pneumocystis pneumonia (PCP) were found among homosexual men in the USA. Human immunodeficiency virus (HIV) was identified as the cause of AIDS in 1983. Infection is transmitted by **sexual intercourse**, by **perinatal transmission** (mother to child transmission in utero, during delivery or by breast feeding) and by exposure to **infected blood** (transfusion of infected blood products, intravenous drug users, needle stick injuries in health care workers).

Epidemiology

It is estimated that since the first case of AIDS was recognised more than 25 years ago about 65 million people have been infected with HIV and 25 million have died of AIDS. The pandemic is worst in sub-Saharan Africa and South-East Asia and is growing fastest in Eastern Europe, Russia and Central Asia. AIDS causes more deaths in Africa than any other disease, and as a result of HIV infection the overall life expectancy of the population of parts of Africa has fallen to 40 years. The routes of transmission of HIV are the same worldwide

but the relative importance of different modes of transmission differs according to the region. Worldwide **heterosexual** transmission accounts for 85% of cases and women comprise half of those infected with HIV. Most HIV infections in Africa are contracted heterosexually, but **mother-to-child** transmission is also an important route of infection and may occur *in utero*, **during delivery** or through **breast feeding. Homosexual** transmission is more common in South-East Asia, Europe, USA and Australia. Transmission associated with **intravenous drug misuse** is common in parts of South-East Asia and Central and South America.

In the UK and Europe the epidemic initially mainly affected homosexual men but now about 30% of new infections have been transmitted heterosexually, and particularly affect those who have recently arrived from a country with a high prevalence of HIV. There is some evidence of a resurgence of HIV infection among homosexual men in the USA, some European countries and Australia apparently because of reduced use of 'safe sex' practices (e.g. condoms) due to complacency arising from the success of anti-retroviral therapy. The treatment of **haemophiliacs** with Factor VIII concentrates derived from large numbers of donors led to a high incidence of HIV infection. Routine testing for HIV in donated blood in the developed countries has stopped transmission of infection in blood products and transfusions.

The global pandemic of HIV infection poses an enormous challenge to the international community, raising complex issues of poverty, politics, health care resources and inequalities in access to modern medicines.

HIV infection

HIV is a retrovirus which has a high affinity for the CD4 molecule of T-lymphocytes. After **binding to the CD4 receptor** the virus penetrates the cell wall and initiates a cycle of **viral replication** within the cell. The replication of retroviruses is driven by the enzyme **reverse transcriptase** which translates the single-stranded viral RNA back to double-stranded DNA—hence the term 'retro' or 'reverse'. The viral DNA is **integrated** into the genome of the cell by the viral enzyme, integrase, and this provirus is then propagated in subsequent generations after each round of cell division. The provirus may remain silent during the lifetime of the cell or be **transcribed**, producing new viral particles which form buds on the cell membrane. The transcription of the provirus is controlled by various proteins derived from the virus itself and from the host cell. On death of the T-cell the virus is released and taken up by new cells, **propagating** infection further. HIV infection results in a progressive fall in the number and function of CD4 T-lymphocytes. The pace at which immunodeficiency develops and the susceptibility to opportunistic infections is reflected in the **CD4 lymphocyte count**. It is possible to measure the HIV replication rate by measuring plasma concentrations of HIV RNA, and this is often referred to as the '**viral load**'.

The average time from initial infection with HIV to the development of AIDS is about 10–12 years. After primary infection with HIV there is an asymptomatic period of about 4 weeks. Then many patients will suffer a 2–3-week **seroconversion illness** which resembles glandular fever with malaise, arthralgia, lymphadenopathy, headache, rashes and fever. This phase is associated with high levels of viraemia, and towards the end of this phase antibodies to HIV are detectable. The virus then becomes mainly localised in lymphoid tissue and the disease enters a chronic symptomless phase. **Persistent generalised lymphadenopathy** may develop. Some patients develop symptoms such as malaise, weight loss and fevers which are caused by HIV infection but not the consequence of opportunistic infections. The term '**AIDS**' is usually used when an HIV-seropositive patient develops certain major opportunistic infections (e.g. PCP, *Mycobacterium avium–intracellulare*), defined malignancies (e.g. Kaposi's sarcoma, non-Hodgkin's lymphoma) or when the CD4 count falls below $200/mm^3$.

Highly active anti-retroviral therapy (Table 8.1)

Highly active anti-retroviral therapy (HAART) became available from 1996 onwards and has resulted in a dramatic decline in the rate of progression of patients from HIV infection to AIDS, and in AIDS-related mortality in the developed countries. These drugs are expensive and are largely not available to the millions of patients with HIV infection in the developing world. Four classes of anti-retroviral drugs are currently available (Table 8.1). Reverse transcriptase catalyses the conversion of single-stranded HIV RNA to double-stranded DNA, which is incorporated into the nucleus of the CD4 cell. **Nucleoside reverse transcriptase inhibitors** block the action of this enzyme and are also incorporated into the DNA sequence causing DNA chain termination. The **non-nucleoside reverse transcriptase inhibitors** bind to reverse transcriptase inhibiting enzyme activity. **Protease inhibitors** block the HIV protease enzyme which is responsible for processing proteins required in the formation of new infective particles. **Fusion inhibitors** block viral entry into cells.

The optimum time for initiation of therapy depends on the **plasma viral load** and **CD4 cell count**, which are monitored throughout treatment. Treatment is typically started when the patient is symptomatic or when the CD4 count has fallen below $300/mm^3$. The development of **drug resistance** is reduced by using **combinations of drugs**. Drug **toxicity** and **interactions** are complex and

Table 8.1 Highly active anti-retroviral drugs.

Drug class	Drugs	Examples of toxicity
Nucleoside reverse transcriptase inhibitors	Zidovudine, stavudine, didanosine, zalcitabine, lamivudine, abacavir	Peripheral neuropathy, rashes, anorexia, nausea, pancreatitis, myalgia, malaise, anaemia
Non-nucleoside reverse transcriptase inhibitors	Efavirenz, nevirapine, delaviridine	Rashes, confusion, nausea, hepatitis, fatigue
Proteinase inhibitors	Amprenavir, indinavir, lopinavir, nelfinavir, ritonavir, saquinavir	Rashes, diarrhoea, renal stones, nausea, pancreatitis
Fusion inhibitors	Enfuviritide	Pancreatitis, neuropathy, dyslipidaemia

treatment regimens must be supervised by specialist HIV physicians. Metabolic effects of anti-retroviral treatment include fat redistribution, insulin resistance and dyslipidaemia. **Adherence** with complex drug regimens can be difficult and patients require **expert support**. Resistance to drugs tends to emerge over time and **sequential therapy**, using different combinations of drugs, may be needed to achieve long-term control of the disease. **Drug interactions** and other drug treatments are important. For example, non-nucleoside drugs and protease inhibitors potentiate the effect of midazolam which should be avoided when these patients are undergoing bronchoscopy (lorazepam can be substituted). Rifampicin, as a P450 inducer, decreases blood levels of anti-retroviral drugs. The restoration of immune function against certain pathogens after starting HAART may provoke an **immune reconstitution inflammatory syndrome** (Table 8.2).

Pulmonary complications of HIV infection (Table 8.2)

Although CD4 T-lymphocytes are the main target of HIV infection, the virus also infects other cells in the body including pulmonary macrophages. A **lymphocytic alveolitis** and **impaired gas diffusion** (reduced transfer factor for carbon monoxide) are found even in asymptomatic patients who do not have evidence of opportunistic infections. There is an increased incidence of **airways disease** and **emphysema** in HIV patients, and this is

probably brought about by pathogenic synergy between HIV infection and smoking, so that smoking cessation should be encouraged. The occurrence of various infections reflects the CD4 T-lymphocyte count and depends on the patient's previous and current exposure to pathogens (e.g. reactivation of previous tuberculosis or re-infection with tuberculosis in areas with a high prevalence, e.g. Africa). As the CD4 T-lymphocyte count falls there is initially an increase in the frequency of infection with common **standard pathogens** (e.g. *Streptococcus pneumoniae*, *Mycobacterium tuberculosis*). Then, as the CD4 count falls below about 200/mm^3, infections with **opportunistic pathogens** (e.g. *Pneumocystis jiroveci*) develop. These are infections which do not usually cause disease in immunocompetent people. In the later stages of AIDS **neoplastic diseases** (e.g. Kaposi's sarcoma, B-cell lymphomas) occur.

Bacterial respiratory infections

Patients with HIV have an increased incidence of respiratory tract infections with **sinusitis, bronchitis, bronchiectasis** and **pneumonia** occurring as a result of standard bacterial pathogens. Infection with *Streptococcus pneumoniae*, *Haemophilus influenzae* and *Staphylococcus aureus* are common, and may precede the diagnosis of HIV infection or the onset of opportunistic infections. Infection with Gram-negative organisms (e.g. *Pseudomonas aeruginosa*) occurs in more advanced disease. The clinical features may be unusual with a higher frequency

Table 8.2 Pulmonary complications of HIV infection.

Infectious diseases
Bacterial infections
  Streptococcus pneumoniae
  Haemophilus influenzae
  Pseudomonas aeruginosa
Tuberculosis
Opportunistic infections
  Fungal
    Pneumocystis jiroveci
    Aspergillus fumigatus
    Candida albicans
  Viral
    Cytomegalovirus
    Herpes simplex
  Mycobacterial
    Mycobacterium avium–intracellulare

Immune reconstitution syndromes
Sarcoid-like syndrome
Paradoxical deterioration of pneumonia

Non-infectious diseases
Neoplastic
  Kaposi's sarcoma
  B-cell lymphoma
  Primary effusion cell lymphoma
Inflammatory
  Lymphocytic alveolitis ($\downarrow T_L co$)
  Non-specific interstitial pneumonitis
  Lymphocytic interstitial pneumonitis
  Airways disease and emphysema
  Primary pulmonary hypertension

of complications such as bacteraemia, abscess formation, cavitation and empyema. Pneumococcal and influenza vaccination may be helpful and sometimes long-term prophylactic antibiotics are used.

Pneumocystis pneumonia

Pneumocystis jiroveci (formerly known as carinii) is a fungus that only causes disease in immunocompromised individuals, and in HIV infection it typically occurs at the stage when the CD4 T-lymphocyte count has fallen to below 200/mm^3. PCP typically presents as a subacute illness over a few weeks with cough, dyspnoea, fever, hypoxaemia, reduced transfer factor for carbon monoxide and bilateral perihilar interstitial infiltrates on chest X-ray (Fig. 8.1).

These clinical features are not specific to PCP and can be caused by a variety of other infections, and more than one pathogen may be present. The chest X-ray may be normal in early PCP and high-resolution computed tomography is more sensitive. Sometimes the radiological features are unusual showing unilateral consolidation, nodules or upper lobe consolidation, for example. Cavitating lesions may occur and pneumothorax is a recognised complication.

The **diagnosis** is usually confirmed by detecting *Pneumocystis jiroveci* using a monoclonal antibody immunofluorescent technique on specimens obtained by **sputum induction** or by bronchoscopy and **bronchoalveolar lavage**. To induce sputum the patient is given 3% hypertonic saline by nebulisation followed by chest physiotherapy. If this test is negative it is usual to proceed to bronchoalveolar lavage whereby a bronchoscope is advanced into a subsegmental bronchus and 60 mL aliquots of warmed sterile saline are instilled and aspirated. More invasive procedures, such as **transbronchial** or **surgical lung biopsy**, are usually only performed in complex cases where the aetiology of lung infiltrates cannot be determined by other tests and where a histological diagnosis is considered essential for guiding treatment decisions.

Treatment of PCP consists of high-dose intravenous **co-trimoxazole** (trimethoprim 20 mg/kg/day and sulfamethoxazole 100 mg/kg/day in four divided doses) subsequently converted to oral therapy, usually continued for 3 weeks. Side-effects (e.g. allergic rashes, nausea, marrow suppression) are common and intravenous **pentamidine** is an alternative treatment. Patients with moderate or severe PCP (e.g. P_{O_2} <9.5 kPa (70 mmHg)) benefit from the addition of **corticosteroids** (e.g. prednisolone 40 mg/day) to reduce the pulmonary inflammatory response. High-flow **oxygen** is often required and use of **continuous positive airway pressure (CPAP)** may reduce the need for **ventilation** in severe cases.

Primary prophylaxis is given to HIV-infected patients whose CD4 T-cell count is <200/mm^3, to prevent first infection. **Secondary prophylaxis** is given to prevent recurrence in patients who have already suffered an episode of PCP. Co-trimoxazole

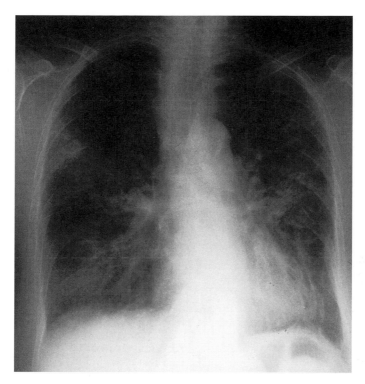

Figure 8.1 Pneumocystis pneumonia. This 28-year-old woman, who was an intravenous drug misuser, presented with fever, dyspnoea and hypoxaemia (P_{O_2} 8.2 kPa (62 mmHg)). Chest X-ray shows diffuse bilateral perihilar and lower zone shadowing. HIV antibody test was positive and CD4 T-lymphocyte count was 100/mm³ (normal 600–1600/mm³). Induced sputum was positive for *Pneumocystis jiroveci* on immunofluorescent monoclonal antibody testing. The patient responded fully to high-dose intravenous co-trimoxazole, prednisolone and oxygen, and she was then commenced on long-term secondary prophylaxis with oral co-trimoxazole 3 days/week. When her pneumocystis pneumonia had been fully treated highly active anti-retroviral therapy was started.

(trimethoprin and sulfamethoxazole) 960 mg given on 3 days/week is the regimen of choice. Nebulised pentamidine given once monthly, atovaquone or a combination of oral pyrimethamine and dapsone are alternatives for patients who cannot tolerate co-trimoxazole. PCP prophylaxis may be stopped in patients who have responded well to HAART with control of viral replication and recovery of CD4 cell counts.

Mycobacterial infection

Mycobacterium tuberculosis (see also Chapter 7)

Patients with HIV infection and impaired CD4 lymphocyte function are highly susceptible to developing **reactivation** of previously acquired latent tuberculosis and to **contracting the disease from an exogenous source**, with rapid **progression to active disease**. In the UK, overlap between the indigenous population with HIV infection (mainly young white men) and the population with tuberculosis (mainly older white people and immigrants from the Indian subcontinent) is low so that only about 5% of patients with HIV infection have tuberculosis. However this may change with the movement of people to the UK from areas of the world with a high prevalence of both HIV and tuberculosis. Worldwide **many millions of people are co-infected with HIV and tuberculosis**, posing a major problem for the global control of tuberculosis. Early in HIV disease, tuberculosis resembles the typical disease seen in non-HIV patients, with upper lobe consolidation and cavitation. In severely immunocompromised patients the clinical features may be very non-specific with fever, weight loss, malaise, diffuse shadowing on chest X-ray and a high incidence of extrapulmonary disseminated disease. Standard anti-tuberculosis treatment is given using isoniazid, rifampicin, pyrazinamide and ethambutol (see Chapter 7). Bacillus Calmette–Guérin (BCG) vaccination is contraindicated in HIV infection because of the risk of active infection developing with the live attenuated vaccine bacillus in severely immunocompromised patients. Because of their impaired cellular immunity, patients with HIV are very susceptible to contracting and transmitting tuberculosis so that strict isolation precautions are warranted, particularly for patients with multidrug-resistant tuberculosis.

Mycobacterium avium–intracellulare complex

This is an opportunistic mycobacterium which does not usually cause disease in normal subjects but which commonly infects patients with advanced AIDS, particularly when the CD4 count is <100/mm^3. Extrapulmonary disease is more common than pulmonary disease and the diagnosis of disseminated *Mycobacterium avium–intracellulare* complex (MAIC) is usually made when the organism is cultured from blood, bone marrow, lymph node or liver biopsy. The organism is not usually responsive to standard anti-tuberculosis drugs and it is treated with a combination of rifabutin, ethambutol, ciprofloxacin and clarithromycin or azithromycin.

Viral infections

Cytomegalovirus (CMV) infection is common in AIDS, usually causing systemic infection with hepatitis, retinitis, encephalitis and colitis, rather than overt pulmonary infection. CMV is often isolated from the lungs of AIDS patients but it is not always pathogenic, sometimes being present as a commensal. It is treated with ganciclovir. **Epstein–Barr virus**, **adenovirus**, **influenza** and **herpes simplex virus** may cause pneumonia in AIDS patients. Herpes simplex virus is frequently present in the mouth of HIV-infected patients so that its isolation from the respiratory tract often indicates colonisation rather than infection.

Fungal pulmonary infections

Invasive pulmonary infections with *Aspergillus fumigatus* or *Candida albicans* are unusual but may occur late in the course of AIDS. **Cryptococcal** pneumonia may occur as part of a disseminated infection but usually meningoencephalitis dominates the clinical picture. Treatment is with fluconazole, flucytosine and amphotericin. Pulmonary **histoplasmosis** and **coccidioidomycosis** may occur in areas where these fungi are endemic (e.g. USA).

HIV-related neoplasms

Kaposi's sarcoma

This is the most common malignancy in HIV-infected patients. Characteristically, it occurs in HIV-infected homosexual men and it is thought that this may relate to **co-infection with human herpes virus 8**. Pulmonary Kaposi's sarcoma is nearly always accompanied by lesions in the skin or buccal mucosa. Chest X-ray appearances are variable as the tumour may affect the bronchi, lung parenchyma, pleura or mediastinal lymph nodes. At bronchoscopy Kaposi's sarcoma appears as red or purple lesions. The diagnosis is usually made on the basis of the visual appearances in the context of mucocutaneous Kaposi's sarcoma as biopsy of the bronchial lesions is often non-diagnostic and may cause haemorrhage. Anti-retroviral therapy (HAART) may lead to regression of Kaposi's sarcoma but anti-neoplastic chemotherapy (e.g. doxorubicin, paclitaxel) is often needed.

Lymphoma

Late in the course of AIDS, high-grade **B-cell lymphomas** arise. The lungs are often involved as part of multiorgan involvement. **Primary effusion lymphoma** can occur and may present with pleural, pericardial or peritoneal effusions. The response to chemotherapy is often poor.

Interstitial pneumonitis

Patients with HIV infection may develop **non-specific interstitial pneumonitis (NSIP)**. This presents as episodes of dyspnoea with pulmonary infiltrates, reduced gas diffusion and hypoxaemia. Bronchoalveolar lavage is negative for infection and transbronchial biopsy shows evidence of lymphocytic inflammation. It may be a manifestation of direct HIV infection of the lung. It is often self-limiting but prednisolone may be beneficial.

Lymphoid interstitial pneumonitis is usually seen only in children with HIV infection, and the pneumonitis may be part of more widespread lymphocytic infiltration of liver, bone marrow and parotid glands with hypergammaglobulinaemia. Its aetiology is uncertain but it may be related to Epstein–Barr virus co-infection.

Primary pulmonary hypertension (see Chapter 16)

This is a rare complication of HIV infection and may result from the effect of inflammatory mediators and cytokines, produced by infection of the lung with the HIV virus, on the pulmonary circulation.

Immune reconstitution syndromes

When anti-retroviral therapy (HAART) inhibits viral replication there is a corresponding increase in the population of T-cells, enhancement of lymphoproliferative responses and increased 1L-2 receptor expression. These proinflammatory effects may give rise to certain syndromes associated with immune reconstitution. Some patients develop a **sarcoid-like granulomatous disorder** with diffuse opacities on chest X-ray, lymphadenopathy, salivary gland enlargement and elevated serum angiotensin-converting enzyme levels. **Pulmonary hypersensitivity** reactions to anti-retroviral drugs have also been described. **Paradoxical deterioration** of opportunistic pneumonia (e.g. PCP, tuberculosis), despite antibiotic therapy, may occur as the patient mounts an inflammatory response. This may be severe enough to cause acute respiratory failure and requires corticosteroid therapy. In patients presenting with HIV infection and low CD4 counts, opportunistic infections should be sought and treated before starting HAART.

Other immunocompromised patients

There is an increasing number of patients who are severely immunocompromised by a variety of diseases and by use of immunosuppressive drugs. Patients with neutropenia are particularly vulnerable to **bacterial infections** (e.g. *Streptococcus pneumoniae*, Gram-negative bacteria) and invasive **fungal infections** (e.g. *Aspergillus fumigatus*, *Candida albicans*), and patients with depressed T-lymphocyte function are vulnerable to **PCP**, **tuberculosis** and **CMV infection**, for example.

There are three particular situations where profound immunosuppression commonly arises:

1 Patients with cancer receiving **anti-neoplastic chemotherapy**.

2 Patients with inflammatory diseases (e.g. connective tissue diseases, Wegener's granulomatosis, inflammatory bowel disease, etc.) receiving **immunosuppressive drugs** (e.g. corticosteroids, cyclophosphamide, methotrexate, infliximab).

3 **Patients post-organ transplantation** (bone marrow, renal, lung, etc.) receiving immunosuppressive drugs (e.g. ciclosporin, azathioprine).

The problem is often that of a patient with one of these conditions presenting with pulmonary infiltrates on chest X-ray accompanied by dyspnoea and sometimes fever. The infiltrates in these circumstances may be caused by pulmonary involvement by the underlying disease process, a reaction to drug treatment, infection resulting from immunosuppression or to other coincidental disease processes. Treatment is crucially dependent upon accurate diagnosis.

Assessment involves a careful clinical history and examination focusing on the clinical context and clues to aetiology (Table 8.3). Microbiology of sputum, urine and blood may identify specific pathogens. Induced sputum is particularly useful in

Table 8.3 Differential diagnosis of pulmonary infiltrates in immunocompromised patients.

Chest X-ray infiltrates
- Is it the underlying disease?
- Is it a reaction to drugs?
- Is it infection?
- Is it some other disease process?

Disease	*Cancer* (e.g. lymphoma, carcinoma)	*Inflammatory disease* (e.g. rheumatoid disease)	*Organ transplant* (e.g. bone marrow, renal)
	Lymphangitis Lung metastases	Interstitial lung disease	Graft versus host disease
Drugs	Lung fibrosis or pneumonitis (e.g. bleomycin, busulfan, cyclophosphamide, methotrexate, gold, penicillamine)		
Infection	Bacterial or opportunistic infections (PCP, CMV)		
Other process	Pulmonary oedema, haemorrhage, embolism, etc.		

Pulmonary infiltrates

↓   Clinical assessment
         Microbiology of sputum, urine, blood (e.g. TB, bacteria)
         Induced sputum (e.g. PCP)
         Bronchoscopy+ bronchoalveolar lavage (CMV, PCP, TB)
         Transbronchial lung biopsy
         Surgical lung biopsy (histology)

Diagnosis ⟶ **Specific treatments**

CMV, cytomegalovirus; PCP, *pneumocystis* pneumonia; TB, tuberculosis.

diagnosing PCP. If these initial tests are not diagnostic it is often advisable to proceed directly to bronchoscopy with bronchoalveolar lavage for detailed microbiology. Transbronchial lung biopsy is useful in obtaining tissue for histological diagnosis but carries the risk of pneumothorax or haemorrhage. Occasionally, surgical lung biopsy is warranted.

Keypoints

- Patients with HIV are initially vulnerable to lung infections with bacteria (e.g. *Streptococcus pneumoniae*, *Mycobacterium tuberculosis*).
- When the CD4 count falls below 200/mm^3 opportunistic infections (e.g. PCP), develop.
- In the late stages of AIDS, neoplastic complications (e.g. Kaposi's sarcoma, B-cell lymphoma) occur.
- Anti-retroviral treatment has improved survival but sometimes provokes an immune reconstitution inflammatory reaction.

Further reading

Beck JM, Rosen MJ, Peavy HH. Pulmonary complications of HIV infection. *Am J Respir Crit Care Med* 2001; **64**: 2120–6.

Fenton KA, Valdiserri RO. Twenty-five years of HIV/AIDS—United States, 1981–2006. *MMWR Morb Mortality Wkly Rep* 2006; **55**: 585–9.

Masur H. Management of patients with HIV in the intensive care unit. *Proc Am Thorac Soc* 2006; **3**: 96–102.

Thomas CF, Limper AH. Pneumocystis pneumonia. *N Engl J Med* 2004; **350**: 2487–98.

Wolff AJ, O'Donnell E. Pulmonary manifestations of HIV infection in the era of highly active antiretroviral therapy. *Chest* 2001; **120**: 1888–93.

Websites: www.unaids.org
www.aidsinfo.nih.gov
www.aidsmap.com

Chapter 9

Bronchiectasis and lung abscess

Bronchiectasis

Bronchiectasis is a chronic disease characterised by irreversible **dilatation of bronchi** caused by bronchial wall damage resulting from infection and inflammation. These morphological changes are usually accompanied by chronic **suppurative lung disease** with cough productive of purulent sputum.

Pathogenesis

Bronchiectasis represents a particular type of bronchial injury which may result from a number of different underlying disease processes. Damage to the bronchial wall causes disruption of the mucociliary escalator and allows bacteria to adhere to the respiratory epithelium and colonise the lung. **Adherence of bacteria** to the respiratory epithelium often involves specific interactions between adhesive structures on the bacterial membrane and receptors on the mucosal surface. After injury the airway epithelium undergoes a process of repair which involves the spreading, migration and proliferation of epithelial cells. During this process epithelial cells synthesise fibronectin, which is required for cell migration, and integrin, which is important for cell-to-cell adhesion. These fibronectin and integrin epithelial receptors are used by the outer membrane protein of bacteria

such as *Pseudomonas aeruginosa* as sites of bacterial adherence. Thus, key elements in the repair process of epithelium are also major receptors for bacterial adherence. The presence of bacteria at a normally sterile site stimulates an inflammatory response as part of the body's attempt to eradicate infection. However, in bronchiectasis this inflammatory response is ineffective in eradicating infection and a persistent cycle of chronic infection and inflammation ensues resulting in further tissue damage.

Bronchiectasis may be confined to one area of the lung if there is a **local** cause (e.g. bronchial obstruction by a foreign body) or may be **diffuse** if there is a generalised cause (e.g. immunoglobulin deficiency). The walls of the bronchi are infiltrated by inflammatory cells, and are thin and dilated with reduced elastin content. The exact mechanisms giving rise to bronchiectasis are not fully understood but the disease seems to evolve through a vicious circle of steps which may be initiated in a variety of ways (Fig. 9.1):

- **Impaired mucociliary clearance** leads to accumulation of secretions.
- Accumulated secretions predispose to bacterial **infection.**
- Infection provokes an **inflammatory response**, increased mucus production and impaired ciliary function.
- Excessive inflammation causes **tissue damage.**
- Damage to the bronchial wall produces **dilatation of bronchi** and disruption of mucociliary

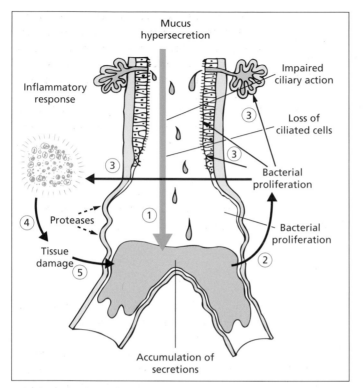

Figure 9.1 Bronchiectasis is often a progressive disease because bronchial damage results in impaired ciliary function with the accumulation of secretions, secondary bacterial infection, a destructive inflammatory response and further bronchial damage in a vicious circle.

clearance, and the vicious circle of injury progresses.

Aetiology (Table 9.1)

Infections

Severe infections are one of the most common causes of bronchial wall damage and bronchiectasis. In childhood, **pertussis (whooping cough)** or **measles** are important causes which are declining in frequency as a result of childhood vaccination programmes. In adults, bronchiectasis may complicate **pneumonia** resulting from virulent organisms such as *Streptococcus pneumoniae*, *Staphylococcus aureus* or *Klebsiella pneumoniae*. Better use of antibiotics has resulted in an overall decline in post-infective bronchiectasis. **Tuberculosis** is still a common cause of bronchiectasis in developing countries. Many adults with **idiopathic** lower lobe bronchiectasis attribute their disease to childhood lung infections.

Table 9.1 Aetiology of bronchiectasis.

Severe infection
   Childhood pertussis
   Bacterial pneumonia
   Recurrent aspiration pneumonia
   Tuberculosis
Bronchial obstruction
   Foreign body (e.g. peanut)
   Bronchial carcinoma
   Lymph node enlargement
Immunodeficient states
   Hypogammaglobulinaemia
   Immunodeficiency as a result of lymphoma
   HIV infection
Allergic bronchopulmonary aspergillosis
Cystic fibrosis (see Chapter 10)
Ciliary dysfunction
   Primary ciliary dyskinesia
   Kartagener's syndrome
Associated diseases
   Ulcerative colitis
   Rheumatoid arthritis
Idiopathic bronchiectasis

Bronchial obstruction

Bronchiectasis may develop in an area of lung obstructed by a bronchial **carcinoma**. In children, inhalation of a **foreign body** (e.g. peanut) may give rise to bronchial obstruction and distal bronchiectasis. **Lymph node enlargement** as part of tuberculosis may compress a bronchus and give rise to bronchiectasis. This particularly occurs in the middle lobe.

Immunodeficiency states

Patients with congenital **hypogammaglobulinaemia** or **selective immunoglobulin deficiencies** usually present with recurrent respiratory tract infections in childhood. Sometimes the diagnosis is not established until adulthood when bronchiectasis may have developed. Serum immunoglobulin levels should be measured in all patients with bronchiectasis because patients with immunoglobulin deficiencies require intravenous immunoglobulin replacement therapy. Immunoglobulin deficiencies may also arise later in life secondary to malignancies such as **lymphoma** or **myeloma**. Patients with **human immunodeficiency virus (HIV) infection** are also susceptible to recurrent bacterial infections and bronchiectasis (see Chapter 8).

Allergic bronchopulmonary aspergillosis (Fig. 9.2)

Aspergillus fumigatus is a ubiquitous fungus which may **colonise** the respiratory tract as an incidental finding without giving rise to symptoms. Patients with lung cavities (e.g. post-tuberculosis or sarcoidosis) may develop an **aspergilloma**, which is a ball of fungal hyphae which appears on X-ray as a mass in the centre of a cavity surrounded by a halo of radiolucency (Fig. 9.3). This is often asymptomatic, but associated inflammation may cause bronchial artery hypertrophy and haemoptysis requiring surgical resection or therapeutic bronchial artery embolisation. **Invasive aspergillosis** (e.g. necrotising pneumonia or fungaemia) occurs in immunocompromised patients (see Chapter 8).

Patients with **asthma** may develop an allergic reaction to *Aspergillus* and demonstrate **precipitating antibodies** to *Aspergillus* in their serum and positive responses to **skin prick tests**. Some of these patients develop **allergic bronchopulmonary aspergillosis** in which there is intense bronchial inflammation with **eosinophilia** and **high IgE** levels in the blood. Eosinophilic infiltrates in the lung give rise to **fleeting X-ray shadows**. Thick **mucus plugs** cause obstruction of small bronchi and give rise to **bronchiectasis** which is usually proximal in location. Treatment requires suppression of the inflammatory immune response by oral prednisolone and high-dose inhaled corticosteroids.

Ciliary dyskinesia

The epithelial cells of the bronchi possess cilia which beat in an organised way so as to move particles in the layer of mucus on their surface upwards and out of the lung. This **mucociliary escalator** is an essential clearance mechanism. Ciliary function is impaired by cigarette smoke and bacterial toxins. Viral infections may cause widespread shedding of ciliated respiratory cells. Bronchial damage of whatever cause often disrupts the mucociliary clearance mechanism impairing the lung defence mechanisms and perpetuating the vicious circle of bronchiectasis.

Primary ciliary dyskinesia is an autosomal recessive condition in which there is an abnormality of the ultrastructure of cilia throughout the body such that they do not beat in a coordinated fashion. Failure of ciliary function in the respiratory tract gives rise to otitis, sinusitis and bronchiectasis. The tail of sperm is also a ciliary structure and males with primary ciliary dyskinesia are subfertile. It is thought that cilia are also responsible for the normal rotation of internal structures in embryonic life so that failure of ciliary function results in random rotation with about 50% of patients having dextrocardia and situs inversus (e.g. appendix in left iliac fossa). Ciliary dyskinesia with situs inversus is known as **Kartagener's syndrome** (Fig. 9.4).

Mucociliary clearance can be assessed by measuring the rate of removal from the lung of an inhaled

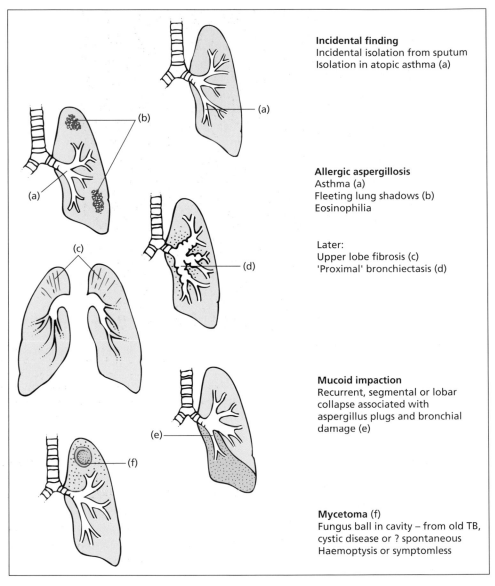

Incidental finding
Incidental isolation from sputum
Isolation in atopic asthma (a)

Allergic aspergillosis
Asthma (a)
Fleeting lung shadows (b)
Eosinophilia

Later:
Upper lobe fibrosis (c)
'Proximal' bronchiectasis (d)

Mucoid impaction
Recurrent, segmental or lobar
collapse associated with
aspergillus plugs and bronchial
damage (e)

Mycetoma (f)
Fungus ball in cavity – from old TB,
cystic disease or ? spontaneous
Haemoptysis or symptomless

Figure 9.2 Summary of the clinical spectrum of *Aspergillus* lung disease.

radiolabelled aerosol. The ultrastructure of cilia can be studied by electron microscopy. Ciliary function can also be studied by microscope photometry which assesses the beat frequency of cilia obtained by brush biopsy of nasal mucosa. A bedside estimate of ciliary function can be obtained by timing the nasal clearance of saccharin. In this test a 1-mm cube of saccharin is placed on the inferior turbinate of the nose. The time from placing the particle to the patient tasting the saccharin is usually less than 30 minutes, and is a measure of nasal ciliary clearance. Nasal mucociliary transport can also be tested by placing a radioisotope, 99 m-Tc-albumin, in the nose and monitoring its movement using a gamma camera. In men, sperm motility may be assessed by microscopy of seminal fluid.

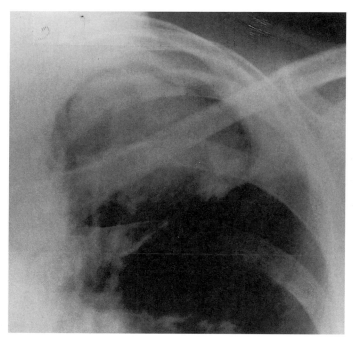

Figure 9.3 This 70-year-old woman had suffered from tuberculosis in the 1950s which had resulted in bilateral apical lung fibrosis and severely impaired lung function (forced expiratory volume in 1 second, 0.5 L; forced vital capacity, 1.1 L). She presented with recurrent major haemoptysis, and chest X-ray showed features characteristic of an aspergilloma with an opacity in the left apex surrounded by a halo of radiolucency. *Aspergillus* hyphae were seen on sputum microscopy and *Aspergillus* precipitins were present in her blood. Tests for carcinoma and tuberculosis were negative. Bronchial arteriography showed marked hypertrophy of the bronchial artery to the left upper lobe and therapeutic embolisation was performed resulting in resolution of the haemoptysis.

Associated diseases

Patients with certain diseases seem to have an increased incidence of bronchiectasis. These diseases include rheumatoid arthritis, ulcerative colitis, Crohn's disease and coeliac disease but the mechanism by which bronchiectasis arises in these diseases is unclear.

Clinical features

The cardinal feature of bronchiectasis is **chronic cough** productive of copious **purulent sputum**. There is considerable variation in the severity of the disease and mild cases are often misdiagnosed as chronic bronchitis. **Haemoptysis** is common and may occasionally be severe, requiring therapeutic embolisation of hypertrophied bronchial arteries to control the bleeding source. Infective exacerbations may be associated with **fever** and **pleuritic pain**.

Chronic severe bronchiectasis may cause **malaise**, **weight loss** and **halitosis** (foul breath). Coarse **crackles** may be audible over affected areas and **clubbing** is sometimes present. Systemic spread of infection (e.g. cerebral abscess) and secondary amyloidosis are now very rare because of control of infection by antibiotics.

Investigations (Fig. 9.5)

A **chest X-ray** may show features of bronchiectasis such as peribronchial thickening, which is evident as parallel tramline shadowing, or cystic dilated bronchi. However, the chest X-ray is often normal in less severe cases and high-resolution **computed tomography (CT)** is the key investigation in confirming the diagnosis and in determining the location and extent of the disease. Bronchography, in which the bronchial tree is

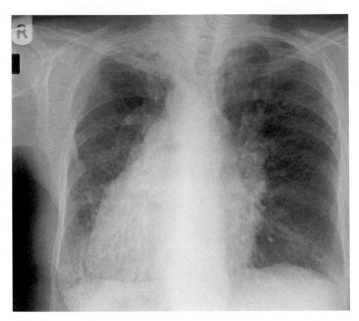

Figure 9.4 This 60-year-old woman has primary ciliary dyskinesia which is an autosomal recessive disorder in which abnormalities of ciliary structure and function give rise to chronic upper and lower respiratory tract infections such as otitis, sinusitis and bronchiectasis. Cilia are also involved in the normal rotation of internal structures in embryonic life and failure of ciliary function results in random rotation such that 50% of these patients have dextrocardia and situs inversus (e.g. heart on the right side and appendix in the left iliac fossa).

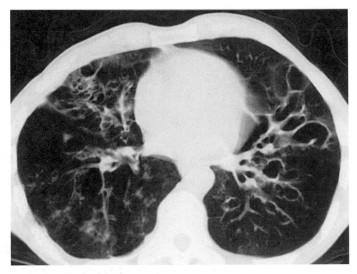

Figure 9.5 This 50-year-old man had suffered pertussis pneumonia at the age of 18 months. He had chronic cough productive of copious purulent sputum isolating *Pseudomonas aeruginosa* on culture. CT showed extensive bilateral bronchiectasis with dilatation of bronchi, cyst formation and patchy peribronchial consolidation. He was treated with postural drainage physiotherapy, salbutamol, long-term nebulised antibiotics (colistin) and intermittent courses of oral ciprofloxacin or intravenous ceftazidime and gentamicin.

outlined by instillation of a radiocontrast dye, has been superseded by CT scanning (Fig. 9.5).

Having confirmed the presence of bronchiectasis, an attempt should be made to diagnose the underlying cause of the bronchiectasis, and further specific tests performed as indicated, for example *Aspergillus* **precipitins** and skin prick tests (allergic bronchopulmonary aspergillosis), **immunoglobulin levels** and IgG subclasses (hypogammaglobulinaemia), **and ciliary function tests** (ciliary dyskinesia). It is important to be aware that the clinical spectrum of cystic fibrosis includes some patients with milder or atypical disease who may not have been diagnosed in early childhood. A **sweat test** and genetic analysis should be performed in patients with diffuse bronchiectasis particularly if other features (e.g. sinusitis, pancreatitis, *Pseudomonas aeruginosa*) are present (see Chapter 10). **Bronchoscopy** is useful in detecting any endobronchial obstruction in cases of localised bronchiectasis. **Sputum microbiology** should be performed to define what infective organisms are present as a guide to antibiotic treatment. **Lung function tests** define the level of any deficit and help determine whether bronchodilator drugs may be helpful.

Treatment

• **Specific treatment** of the underlying cause is rarely possible but relief of endobronchial obstruction (e.g. foreign body) is the key treatment for some patients, intravenous immunoglobulin replacement therapy is essential for patients with hypogammaglobulinaemia, and suppression of the inflammatory response by oral or inhaled corticosteroids is important in allergic aspergillosis.
• **Chest physiotherapy** is the most effective treatment in preventing the accumulation of secretions. Postural drainage (using gravity-assisted positions to aid clearance of secretions from affected areas), percussion and forced expiratory techniques ('huffing') should be guided by a physiotherapist.
• **Antibiotics** are used to suppress chronic infection and to treat exacerbations. High doses are required to penetrate the scarred bronchial mucosa and purulent secretions. The choice of antibiotics is guided by the results of sputum microbiology.

Haemophilus influenzae and *Streptococcus pneumoniae* are common and are usually sensitive to amoxicillin. Antibiotic resistance may develop, and the presence of co-infection with *Moraxella catarrhalis* is usually associated with the production of β-lactamase so that co-amoxiclav or ciprofloxacin may be useful. *Pseudomonas aeruginosa* is common in severe disease and may be treated by oral ciprofloxacin or intravenous anti-pseudomonal antibiotics (e.g. meropenem, ceftazidime, gentamicin). Nebulised antibiotics (e.g. colistin, tobramycin) may be used to suppress chronic *Pseudomonas* infection. Long-term oral antibiotics (e.g. amoxicillin) are sometimes used in severe disease but there is a risk of promoting antibiotic resistance. Anaerobic infections (e.g. *Bacteroides*) are quite common and respond to metronidazole. Long-term treatment with a macrolide antibiotic (e.g. azithromycin) may reduce the frequency of exacerbations of bronchiectasis, possibly by an anti-inflammatory rather than an anti-microbial effect. Pneumococcal and influenza vaccinations are recommended for patients with bronchiectasis.
• **Bronchodilator drugs** (e.g. salbutamol, terbutaline) and an **inhaled steroid** (e.g. beclometasone, budesonide, fluticasone) are indicated where there is associated reversible airways obstruction.
• **Surgical excision** is a potential treatment for the few patients who have localised disease and troublesome symptoms. **Lung transplantation** is an option for patients whose disease has progressed to respiratory failure.

Lung abscess (Fig. 9.6)

A lung abscess is a **localised collection of pus within a cavitated necrotic lesion in the lung parenchyma**. The chest X-ray characteristically shows a cavitating lesion containing a fluid level. The patient typically complains of cough with expectoration of large amounts of foul material often accompanied by haemoptysis, fever, weight loss and malaise. It is important to distinguish between a lung abscess and other causes of cavitating lung lesions, such as a squamous cell carcinoma, and bronchoscopy or percutaneous fine-needle aspiration of the lesion may be required.

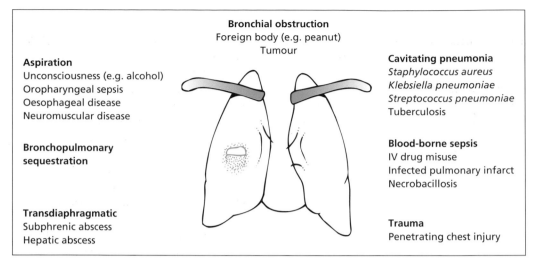

Figure 9.6 Aetiology of lung abscess.

The infection giving rise to a lung abscess may arise via a number of routes. Oropharyngeal **aspiration** is the most common cause and occurs in states of unconsciousness (e.g. alcohol excess, epilepsy, anaesthesia), and where there is dysphagia as a result of oesophageal or neuromuscular disease. Infection of the upper airways (e.g. sinusitis, dental abscess) may be an important source of bacteria, and anaerobic organisms (e.g. *Bacteroides*, *Streptococcus milleri*) are common. Infection may arise distal to **bronchial obstruction** caused by a tumour or foreign body (e.g. inhaled peanut). The centre of an area of destructive **pneumonia** may break down to form a lung abscess particularly when the pneumonia results from *Staphylococcus aureus* or *Klebsiella pneumoniae*. Tuberculosis may present as a lung abscess. **Blood-borne** infection may occur by intravenous injection of infected material by drug addicts. Pulmonary emboli may cause pulmonary infarction, with secondary infection giving rise to an abscess. Penetrating **chest trauma** is an unusual cause of lung abscess. **Transdiaphragmatic** spread of infection may occur from a subphrenic abscess (e.g. post-cholecystectomy) or a hepatic abscess (e.g. amoebic abscess).

Drainage of pus from the abscess cavity is a key aspect of treatment. This can often be achieved by bronchial drainage using postural drainage physiotherapy. Sometimes percutaneous drainage is achieved by positioning a catheter drainage tube under radiological guidance. Prolonged **antibiotic** therapy is given in accordance with the likely organism and the results of microbiology tests (e.g. metronidazole for anaerobic infections). **Surgical excision** of the abscess cavity is sometimes required where medical treatment fails.

Necrobacillosis

Necrobacillosis (Lemière's disease) is an unusual cause of lung abscess which is associated with a very characteristic clinical picture first described by Lemière. Typically, a young adult develops a **severe sore throat** with **cervical adenopathy** because of infection with the anaerobe, *Fusobacterium necrophorum*. This is associated with a local venulitis followed by a **septicaemic illness** with haematogenous spread of infection. The lungs are frequently involved with multiple **abscesses** forming, often with a **pleural empyema** and evidence of infection elsewhere (e.g. **septic arthritis**, **osteomyelitis**). Prolonged anaerobic blood culture is required to identify the organism, which is sensitive to metronidazole.

Bronchopulmonary sequestration

Bronchopulmonary sequestration is a congenital anomaly in which an **area of lung is not connected to the bronchial tree** (i.e. 'sequestered') and has an **anomalous blood supply** usually from the aorta. If infection develops in the sequestration it often progresses to an abscess because of lack of drainage to the bronchial tree. Surgical resection is required but pre-operative bronchial arteriography is necessary to identify the anomalous blood supply.

Keypoints

- Bronchiectasis is characterised by permanent dilatation of bronchi due to bronchial damage caused by infection and inflammation.
- High-resolution CT is the key investigation in confirming the diagnosis.
- Investigations for specific causes of bronchiectasis include sweat tests (cystic fibrosis), immunoglobulin levels (hypogammaglobulinaemia), *Aspergillus* preciptins (allergic aspergillosis) and ciliary tests (primary ciliary dyskinesia).
- Treatment involves chest physiotherapy, antibiotics, inhaled bronchodilators and corticosteroids, and specific treatment of any underlying cause.
- A lung abscess is a localised collection of pus within a cavitated necrotic lesion in the lung parenchyma.

Further reading

Barker AF. Bronchiectasis. *N Engl J Med* 2002; **346**: 1383–93.

Chapel HM. Consensus on diagnosis and management of primary antibody deficiencies. *BMJ* 1994; **308**: 581–5.

Davies G, Wilson R. Prophylactic antibiotic treatment of bronchiectasis with azithromycin. *Thorax* 2004; **59**: 540–1.

DeBoeck K, Wilschanski M, Castellani C et al. Cystic fibrosis: terminology and diagnostic algorithms. *Thorax* 2006; **61**: 627–35.

Lavery K, Bradley JM, Elborn JS. Bronchiectasis: challenges in diagnosis and management. *Int J Respir Care* 2005: 92–8.

Noone PG, Leigh MW, Sannuti A et al. Primary ciliary dyskinesia: diagnostic and phenotypic features. *Am J Respir Crit Care Med* 2004; **169**: 459–67.

Ooi GC, Khong PL, Chan-Yeung M et al. High-resolution CT quantification of bronchiectasis: clinical and functional correlation. *Radiology* 2002; **225**: 663–72.

The primary ciliary dyskinesia family support group. www.p-c-d.org.uk

Tsang KW, Tan KC, Ho PL et al. Inhaled fluticasone in bronchiectasis: a 12 month study. *Thorax* 2005; **60**: 239–43.

Chapter 10

Cystic fibrosis

Introduction

Cystic fibrosis is the most common potentially lethal inherited disease of Caucasians. **It affects about 1 in 2500 live births** in the UK and is inherited in an autosomal recessive manner. About **1 in 25 of the population is a carrier** of the disease.

The basic defect

Cystic fibrosis is a result of a defect in a gene on the long arm of chromosome 7 which codes for a 1480-amino-acid protein, named **cystic fibrosis transmembrane conductance regulator (CFTR)**. More than 1000 mutations of this gene have been identified but the most common is designated ΔF508, in which mutation of a single codon of the gene results in the loss of phenylalanine ('delta F') at position 508 of the protein. CFTR functions as a **chloride channel** in the membrane of epithelial cells and the primary physiological defect in cystic fibrosis is reduced chloride conductance at epithelial membranes, most notably in the respiratory, gastrointestinal, pancreatic, hepatobiliary and reproductive tracts. In sweat ducts, failure of reabsorption of chloride ions results in elevated concentrations of chloride and sodium in the sweat, a characteristic feature of the disease and the basis for the sweat test used in diagnosis.

Lungs

In the bronchial mucosa reduced chloride secretion and increased sodium reabsorption results in **secretions of abnormal viscosity** with reduced water content of the airway surface liquid and reduced depth of the periciliary fluid, predisposing to adherence and reduced clearance of bacteria. The **high salt content** of airway surface fluid **inactivates defensins** which are naturally occurring antimicrobial peptides on the epithelial surface. There is some evidence that the CFTR also has a role in the normal uptake and processing of *Pseudomonas aeruginosa* from the respiratory tract. Patients with cystic fibrosis also have abnormal mucus glycoproteins which act as binding sites such that **bacteria adhere to the mucosa** and proliferate. Thus, the gene defect results in dysfunction of CFTR and predisposes to severe chronic lung infection by a variety of mechanism at the cellular level. The inflammatory response is unable to clear the infection and a vicious cycle of **infection** and **inflammation** develops, progressing to lung damage, **bronchiectasis**, **respiratory failure** and **death**.

Gastrointestinal tract

In the **pancreas** the abnormal ion transport results in the plugging and obstruction of ductules with progressive destruction of the gland. The pancreatic enzymes (e.g. lipase) fail to reach the small intestine and this results in **malabsorption** of fats with steatorrhoea and failure to gain weight. Progressive destruction of the endocrine pancreas may cause **diabetes**. Abnormalities of bile secretion and absorption cause an increased incidence of **gallstones** and **biliary cirrhosis**. Sludging and desiccation of intestinal contents probably accounts for the occurrence of **meconium ileus** (neonatal intestinal obstruction) in about 10% of babies with cystic fibrosis, and for the development of **distal intestinal obstruction syndrome** (meconium ileus equivalent) in older children and adults.

Clinical features (Fig. 10.1)

Infants and young children

About 10% of children with cystic fibrosis present at birth with **meconium ileus**, a form of intestinal obstruction caused by inspissated viscid faecal material resulting from lack of pancreatic enzymes and from reduced intestinal water secretion. More than half of children affected by cystic fibrosis have obvious malabsorption by the age of 6 months with **failure to thrive** associated with abdominal distension and copious offensive stools from **steatorrhoea** as a result of malabsorbed fat. **Rectal prolapse** occasionally occurs. Recurrent **respiratory infections** rapidly become a prominent feature with cough, sputum production and wheeze. Neonatal screening programmes are being introduced which allow the early diagnosis of cystic fibrosis, before the onset of symptoms and complications.

Older children and adults

Respiratory disease (Fig. 10.2)

Persistent cough and purulent sputum characterise the development of **bronchiectasis**. Progressive lung damage is associated with the development of digital clubbing and progressive **airways obstruction**, sometimes associated with wheeze. Serial measurements of forced expiratory volume in 1 second (FEV_1) give an indication of the severity and progression of the disease. Some patients show a

significant asthmatic component with reversible airways obstruction and some develop colonisation of the bronchi by *Aspergillus fumigatus* and may show features of allergic bronchopulmonary aspergillosis (see Chapter 9). Initially, the typical organisms isolated in sputum cultures are *Staphylococcus aureus*, *Haemophilus influenzae* and *Streptococcus pneumoniae*. By teenage years many have become infected with mucoid strains of *Pseudomonas aeruginosa*. *Burkholderia cepacia* complex is a group of Gram-negative plant pathogens which cause onion rot. It was initially thought that these organisms were not pathogenic to humans but in the 1980s it became apparent that patients with cystic fibrosis were vulnerable to these bacteria and that infection could spread from patient to patient in an epidemic way, particularly amongst children with cystic fibrosis in close social contact in holiday camps, for example. The clinical course of patients with *Burkholderia cepacia complex* infection is very variable but some show an accelerated rate of decline in lung function and some develop a fulminant necrotising pneumonia, the so-called 'cepacia syndrome' (Fig. 10.3). It is now recognised that there are many different strains of this bacterium but *Burkholderia cenocepacia* genomovar III is associated with the worst prognosis. Because of the potential for transmission of infection between patients with cystic fibrosis it is now standard practice to segregate patients with different infections such that they attend different clinics and wards, and social contact between patients with cystic fibrosis is discouraged.

As the cycle of infection and inflammation progresses, lung damage worsens with deteriorating airways obstruction, destruction of lung parenchyma, impairment of gas exchange and the development of **hypoxaemia**, **hypercapnia** and **cor pulmonale**. The persistent pulmonary inflammation provokes hypertrophy of the bronchial arteries, and **haemoptysis** becomes common. Occasionally, when severe bleeding occurs, therapeutic embolisation of the bronchial arteries may be required. **Pneumothorax** occurs in about 5–10% of patients with advanced disease and may require prompt tube drainage. Pleurodesis may be required for recurrent pneumothoraces but this should be performed with

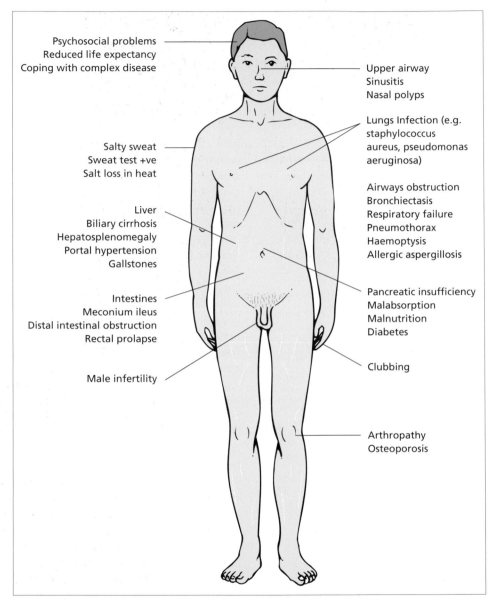

Psychosocial problems
Reduced life expectancy
Coping with complex disease

Upper airway
Sinusitis
Nasal polyps

Lungs Infection (e.g.
staphylococcus
aureus, pseudomonas
aeruginosa)

Salty sweat
Sweat test +ve
Salt loss in heat

Airways obstruction
Bronchiectasis
Respiratory failure
Pneumothorax
Haemoptysis
Allergic aspergillosis

Liver
Biliary cirrhosis
Hepatosplenomegaly
Portal hypertension
Gallstones

Intestines
Meconium ileus
Distal intestinal obstruction
Rectal prolapse

Pancreatic insufficiency
Malabsorption
Malnutrition
Diabetes

Male infertility

Clubbing

Arthropathy
Osteoporosis

Figure 10.1 Clinical features of cystic fibrosis. Cystic fibrosis is a multisystem disease resulting from mutations of the gene which codes for a protein, CFTR, which functions as a chloride channel on epithelial membranes. Failure of chloride conductance results in abnormal secretions and organ damage in the respiratory, pancreatic, hepatobiliary, gastrointestinal and reproductive tracts.

care so as not to compromise future potential lung transplantation.

Gastrointestinal disease

About 85% of patients with cystic fibrosis have **pancreatic insufficiency** with **malabsorption of** fat because of lack of lipase. Unless these patients receive adequate pancreatic enzyme supplements they develop steatorrhoea with frequent bulky offensive stools and failure to gain weight. Progressive destruction of the endocrine pancreas is manifest by an increasing incidence of **diabetes**

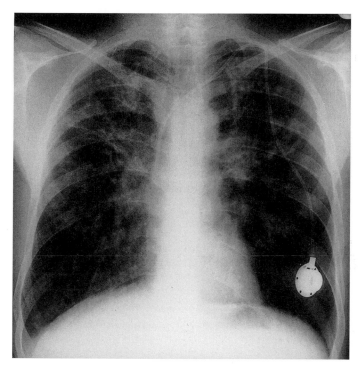

Figure 10.2 Chest X-ray of this 37-year-old man with cystic fibrosis shows hyperinflation, peribronchial thickening, cystic bronchiectasis and perihilar fibrosis. A Portacath central venous system is in place with the access port situated subcutaneously in the left lower chest. He has chronic *Pseudomonas aeruginosa* infection and receives about three courses of intravenous ceftazidime and tobramycin at home each year. His FEV_1 is 1.5 L (42% of predicted) and his general condition and lung function have remained stable over the last 5 years on treatment including long-term nebulised colistin, nebulised deoxyribonuclease, physiotherapy and nutritional supplements.

as these patients get older. A variety of **hepatobiliary abnormalities** occur including fatty liver, gallstones and focal biliary fibrosis, and about 5% of patients develop multinodular cirrhosis with hepatosplenomegaly, portal hypertension, oesophageal varices and liver failure. **Distal intestinal obstruction syndrome** (meconium ileus equivalent) (Fig. 10.4) results from inspissated fatty semi-solid faecal material obstructing the terminal ileum. A number of factors contribute to the development of this complication including malabsorption of fat, disordered intestinal motility and dehydrated intestinal contents resulting from defective intestinal chloride transport. The clinical features vary depending on the severity of the obstruction. Typically, the patient suffers recurrent episodes of colicky abdominal pain and constipation, and there is often a palpable mass in the right

iliac fossa. In severe cases complete intestinal obstruction may develop with abdominal distension, vomiting and multiple fluid levels in distended small bowel on an erect X-ray of abdomen. It is treated by a balanced intestinal lavage solution (e.g. Klean-Prep®) which is taken orally or by nasogastric tube. The radiocontrast Gastrografin (sodium diatrizoate) may also be used as this agent has detergent properties which allow it to penetrate the inspissated fatty material and its hypertonicity then draws fluid into the faecal bolus. Other measures include rehydration, stool softeners (e.g. lactulose) and *N*-acetylcysteine which probably acts by cleaving disulphide bonds in the mucoprotein faecal bolus. Prevention of recurrence requires adequate pancreatic enzyme supplements, avoidance of dehydration and sometimes use of laxatives.

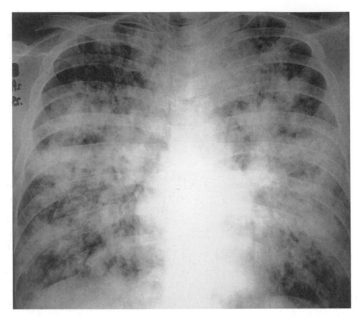

Figure 10.3 'Cepacia syndrome': chest X-ray of this 23-year-old man with cystic fibrosis shows the typical appearance of 'cepacia syndrome' with fulminant bilateral necrotising pneumonia. He had acquired *Burkholderia cenocepacia* genomovar III infection 7 years previously during an outbreak of infection amongst patients with cystic fibrosis attending a holiday camp. His lung function showed an accelerated rate of decline in the years after infection and he then developed a severe exacerbation that failed to respond to treatment and progressed to a fatal fulminant pneumonia over a 2-week period.

Other complications

Nearly all **male patients are infertile** because of congenital bilateral absence of the vas deferens. The exact mechanism by which this complication occurs is not known but it has been suggested that it may result from resorption of the vas deferens after it has become plugged with viscid secretions in foetal life. Techniques such as microsurgical sperm aspiration from the epididymis or testes, with in vitro fertilisation by intracytoplasmic sperm injection can facilitate parenthood for men. Females have near normal fertility although some abnormalities of cervical mucus are present. **Pregnancy** places additional burdens on the mother's health and is sometimes associated with a deterioration in the disease because of increased nutritional stress and impaired bronchial clearance. However, the main risk is of the mother failing to maintain all aspects of her own treatment as she focuses on the care of the baby.

Upper airway involvement causes troublesome **sinusitis** and **nasal polyps**. Cystic fibrosis **arthropathy** probably results from the deposition in joints of antigen–antibody complexes produced by the immune response to bacterial lung infections. Vasculitic **rashes** may also occur. In hot weather, patients with cystic fibrosis are at risk of developing **heat prostration** as a result of excess loss of salt in sweat. As these patients are living longer, a number of other complications are being described such as **osteoporosis** and **amyloidosis**. Patients with cystic fibrosis face major **social and emotional stresses** relating to their reduced life expectancy, outlook for employment, ability to form relationships and undertake marriage and their general capacity to cope with a complex disease and its treatment.

Diagnosis

The diagnosis of cystic fibrosis is based upon the demonstration of **elevated sweat chloride** concentrations on a sweat test, in association with **characteristic clinical features** such as recurrent respiratory infections or evidence of pancreatic

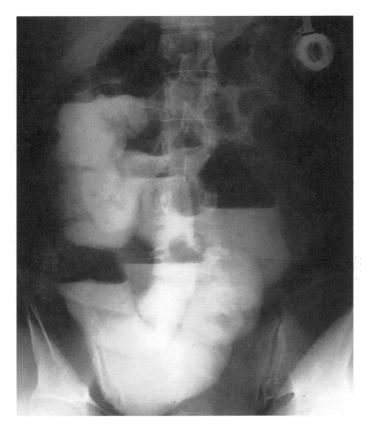

Figure 10.4 Meconium ileus equivalent. This 31-year-old woman with cystic fibrosis was admitted to hospital complaining of abdominal distension, colicky pain and constipation. A mass of inspissated faecal material was palpable in the right iliac fossa. Erect abdominal X-ray (after taking Gastrografin) shows distended loops of small bowel containing multiple fluid levels. A diagnosis of meconium ileus equivalent (distal intestinal obstruction syndrome) was made and she was treated with Gastrografin (orally and by enema), *N*-acetylcysteine orally, intravenous fluids, followed by flushing of the bowel using balanced intestinal lavage solution.

insufficiency. Nowadays the diagnosis is usually confirmed by the demonstration of **two known cystic fibrosis mutations** (e.g. ΔF508/ΔF508) on DNA analysis. It is possible to detect abnormal chloride conductance directly by measuring the potential difference of the nasal mucosa although this is a specialist research technique.

Sweat testing

In cystic fibrosis the ion-transport defect results in a failure to reabsorb chloride ions from the sweat, so that elevated sweat chloride and sodium concentrations are a characteristic feature of the disease. Sweating is induced by **pilocarpine**

iontophoresis, the sweat is collected on filter paper and then analysed for sodium and chloride. Pilocarpine is placed on the skin of the forearm and a small electrical current is passed across it to enhance its penetration of the skin and stimulation of the sweat ducts. Meticulous technique is required to avoid evaporation of secretions or contamination. A sweat flow rate of at least 100 μL/min is required for accurate analysis and sweat chloride levels above 60 mmol/L on repeated tests are abnormal.

DNA analysis

The discovery of the cystic fibrosis gene in 1989 led to the development of **genotyping as an aid to**

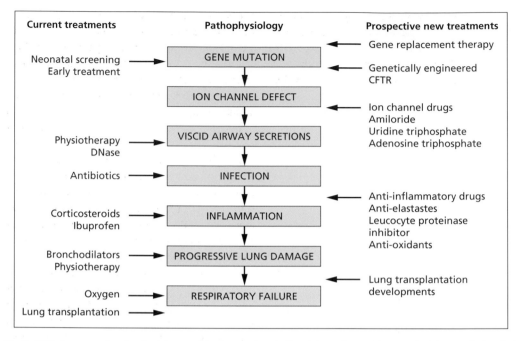

Figure 10.5 Summary of pathophysiology and treatment of cystic fibrosis lung disease. The genetic defect results in a lack of CFTR and abnormal chloride transport in airway epithelium. The resultant viscid secretions predispose to the acquisition and persistence of bacterial infection. The inflammatory response is unable to clear infection and a vicious cycle of infection and inflammation causes bronchiectasis and progressive lung damage, leading to respiratory failure and death, over a median period of 30 years. Key elements of treatment at all stages of the disease are nutrition, antibiotics, chest physiotherapy and psychosocial support. A variety of currently available and prospective treatments target the different pathophysiological stages of the disease to improve the outlook for patients with cystic fibrosis.

diagnosis. Genotyping can also be used to detect **carrier status**, and can be applied to chorionic villus biopsy material for **antenatal diagnosis**. However, there are more than 1000 mutations of the cystic fibrosis gene currently identified and it is only possible to test for the more common mutations so that it can be difficult to exclude cystic fibrosis resulting from rare mutations. DNA analysis has established the diagnosis in some individuals with only mild clinical features, and this has extended our knowledge of the clinical spectrum of the disease to include some very rare older, less severely affected patients. Affected individuals have two gene mutations, one inherited from each of their parents. Carriers of the disease have only one abnormal gene, and do not show any evidence of the disease.

Screening

Early diagnosis of cystic fibrosis allows specific treatment to be commenced rapidly, and this is associated with an improved prognosis. Infants with cystic fibrosis have elevated serum **immunoreactive trypsin activity**. This can be measured on a single dried blood spot obtained on a Guthrie card as part of the neonatal screening programme for diseases such as phenylketonuria and hypothyroidism.

Treatment (Fig. 10.5)

Cystic fibrosis is a complex multisystem disease, and skills from several disciplines are needed in treating these patients. The optimal use of currently available treatments and the introduction of new treatments is best achieved by concentrating the care of these patients in regional **specialist centres**. The basic elements of treatment comprise clearance of bronchial secretions by **physiotherapy**, treatment of pulmonary infection by **antibiotics** and correction of nutritional deficits by use of **pancreatic enzyme supplements** and **dietary support**. Patients and their families require continuous encouragement and support in coping with this complex disease. The Cystic Fibrosis Trust acts as a focus of **information and support**, and coordinates fund raising for research.

Chest physiotherapy

The viscid purulent sputum results in airways obstruction, and clearance of airway secretions by chest physiotherapy is important at all stages of the disease. A variety of techniques can be used including **postural drainage** (using gravity-assisted positions to aid drainage), chest **percussion** and **positive expiratory pressure devices** to aid dislodgement and expectoration of sputum from the peripheral airways. As patients mature it is important that they learn to perform bronchial clearance themselves. The 'active cycle of breathing technique' is often effective and popular with adult patients. This involves a **cycle of breathing control**, thoracic expansion exercises and the **forced expiratory technique** ('huffing') which releases secretions from peripheral bronchi. Exercise is an excellent adjunct to physiotherapy but should not replace it.

Antibiotics

Children with cystic fibrosis should be **immunised** against pertussis and measles as part of the childhood vaccination programme, and should receive annual influenza vaccination thereafter. They should avoid contact with people with respiratory infections and avoid inhalation of cigarette smoke. A variety of antibiotic strategies are used. *Staphylococcus aureus* is a major pathogen in the disease from early childhood and long-term continuous **flucloxacillin** is often used to suppress this infection.

Further oral antibiotics are given during exacerbations in accordance with sputum cultures and sensitivity testing. Common pathogens include *Haemophilus influenzae* and *Streptococcus pneumoniae* which are usually sensitive to **amoxicillin**.

Infection with *Pseudomonas aeruginosa* becomes an increasing problem as children get older, and an important strategy in antibiotic therapy is to postpone for as long as possible the colonisation of the airways by this organism. Frequent sputum cultures are performed and intensive anti-pseudomonal antibiotic therapy is given when the organism is first isolated. This often comprises an **initial prolonged course of oral ciprofloxacin** and **nebulised colistin or tobramycin**. If this does not eradicate infection then **intravenous anti-pseudomonal antibiotics** are recommended. Eventually, chronic infection with *Pseudomonas aeruginosa* becomes established. Attempts at suppressing the effects of this infection involve long-term use of **nebulised antibiotics** such as colistin or tobramycin with additional courses of intravenous anti-pseudomonal antibiotics during infective exacerbations or when there is a decline in lung function. Usually an aminoglycoside (e.g. gentamicin, tobramycin) is given in combination with a third-generation cephalosporin (e.g. ceftazidime) or a modified penicillin (e.g. piperacillin). Treatment is usually given for 14 days and high doses are required to achieve adequate penetration of antibiotics into scarred bronchial mucosa because patients with cystic fibrosis have increased renal clearance of antibiotics.

Intravenous antibiotic treatment is often given **at home** by the patient after training. Where venous access is difficult a totally implanted central venous device can be inserted (e.g. Portacath). This comprises a central venous cannula connected to a subcutaneous port which is accessed by inserting a special non-cutting needle through the skin and the diaphragm of the subcutaneous chamber.

Burkholderia cepacia complex organisms are usually resistant to many of the commonly used anti-pseudomonal antibiotics such as colistin, ciprofloxacin and aminoglycosides, but are often sensitive to ceftazidime or meropenem.

Bronchodilator medication

Some patients with cystic fibrosis have a reversible component to their airways obstruction, and benefit from bronchodilator drugs (e.g. salbutamol, terbutaline) and inhaled steroids (e.g. beclometasone, budesonide, fluticasone).

Deoxyribonuclease

The sputum of patients with cystic fibrosis contains high levels of DNA which is derived from the nuclei of decaying neutrophils. This makes the sputum very viscid and difficult to expectorate. Recombinant human deoxyribonuclease (Dnase/dornase alfa) is a genetically engineered enzyme which cleaves DNA. This treatment can be administered by nebulisation and improves the lung function and reduces the number of exacerbations in some patients.

Anti-inflammatory drugs

The inflammatory response is unable to eradicate infection and contributes to the progressive lung damage. Corticosteroid drugs (e.g. **prednisolone**) may have a beneficial effect but their use is limited by adverse effects. High-dose **ibuprofen** may also be useful in reducing lung injury by inhibiting the migration and activation of neutrophils. **Macrolide antibiotics** (e.g. azithromycin) have recently been shown to improve lung function in patients with cystic fibrosis. This seems to be due to an anti-inflammatory effect by suppression of inflammatory cytokines, reducing neutrophil function and impairing biofilm formation around Pseudomonas aeruginosa.

Nutrition

Pancreatic enzyme supplements (e.g. Creon, Pancrease, Nutrizym) are taken with each meal and with snacks containing fat. Enteric-coated preparations protect the lipase from inactivation by gastric acid, and use of antacid medication (e.g.

omeprazole, lansoprazole) may improve effectiveness. The dose of enzyme is adjusted according to the dietary intake to optimise weight gain and growth and to control steatorrhoea. Use of high doses of pancreatic enzymes has been associated with the development of strictures of the ascending colon—so-called 'fibrosing colonopathy'—in a small number of children so that it is recommended that the dose of lipase should not exceed 10 000 U/kg/day. Supplements of **fat-soluble vitamins** (A, D, E) are routinely given.

Patients with cystic fibrosis suffer from nutritional deficiencies as a result of malabsorption and the increased energy requirements resulting from increased energy expenditure because of chronic lung infection. Most patients with cystic fibrosis require 120–150% of the recommended daily calorie intake for normal individuals, so that healthy eating for a patient with cystic fibrosis includes **high-energy foods** and frequent snacks between main meals. **Dietary supplements** (e.g. Fortisip, Scandishake) are useful when factors such as anorexia limit intake. In advanced disease **nocturnal enteral feeding** of high-energy formulas, through a nasogastric tube or gastrostomy, may be required.

Advanced disease

The clinical course of cystic fibrosis is very variable but an FEV_1 of less then 30% of the predicted value, for example, is associated with a 50% 2-year mortality rate. An awareness of the stage of the disease and the likely prognosis assists in planned management. Oxygen saturation should be measured by oximetry at each clinic visit in patients with advanced disease and when hypoxaemia develops domiciliary **oxygen** may alleviate the complications of respiratory failure. **Lung transplantation** is the main option to be considered for patients with advanced disease but the lack of donor organs severely limits the use of this treatment (see Chapter 21). Some patients will opt for a **palliative care** approach avoiding unpleasant interventions and focusing on measures which alleviate symptoms. Death is usually peaceful after a short coma due to ventilatory failure.

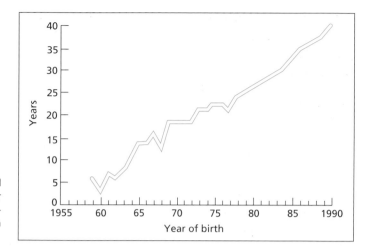

Figure 10.6 Projected median survival of patients with cystic fibrosis by year of birth from 1959 to 1990. (Reproduced with permission from Elborn et al., 1991.)

Prognosis (Fig. 10.6)

The prognosis of patients with cystic fibrosis has improved dramatically over the years. In the 1950s, survival beyond 10 years was unusual. Now the median survival is about 30 years and it is predicted to be at least 40 years for children born in the 1990s. There are now about 6250 patients with cystic fibrosis in the UK, of whom 40% are adults (aged 16 or over). Patients entering adulthood with cystic fibrosis face a number of problems, particularly relating to their chronic lung disease and reduced life expectancy (e.g. life insurance, choice of career, relationships, marriage, pregnancy, fertility). The improved survival of patients with cystic fibrosis has been attributed to a combination of factors including improved management of meconium ileus in neonates, earlier diagnosis, better dietary management and pancreatic enzyme supplementation and meticulous attention to physiotherapy and antibiotic treatments in specialist centres. Although cystic fibrosis typically produces severe progressive lung disease there is a wide **clinical spectrum of severity**. Some 'milder mutations' are associated with residual chloride conductance and less severe clinical disease but there is generally a poor correlation between specific gene mutations and clinical manifestations. Environmental factors, therapeutic regimens and additional 'modifier genes' which influence cytokine responses, for

example, are important. Some patients are well and leading relatively normal lives, well into adulthood, and there is a need to adapt treatment to the stage and severity of the disease. With improved survival treatments need to be planned with care over decades to avoid adverse effects (e.g. aminoglycoside nephrotoxicity, antibiotic allergy and resistance) and to prevent long-term complications of the disease (e.g. osteoporosis, diabetic complications)

Prospective treatments

Ongoing refinements of conventional care in specialist centres continue to improve survival rates. **Neonatal screening** offers the prospect of early diagnosis before the onset of symptoms and this allows specific treatments to be commenced rapidly. This has been shown to improve growth and nutritional status in the early years. Nebulised **hypertonic saline** has recently been shown to improve lung function by drawing water into the airways with improved mucus clearance. The identification of the cystic fibrosis gene in 1989 has revolutionised our understanding of the detailed pathophysiology of this disease at the cellular level and offers the prospect of developing treatments directed against the basic underlying defects. Perhaps the most exciting approach is the direct replacement of the defective gene by

gene therapy. The cystic fibrosis gene has been cloned and given to patients in experimental trials using liposomes as gene transfer agents to introduce the gene into epithelial cells. Expression of the gene can be detected by measuring transepithelial potential differences. Although gene transfer and expression have been achieved many practical difficulties have to be overcome before gene therapy can be considered as a clinically effective treatment for patients. **Pharmacological therapies** may be able to improve the function of mutant CFTR by improving its movement to the cell membrane and by stimulating its function. A further approach is to attempt to correct the ion channel defect by stimulating alternative chloride channels or inhibiting sodium channels. Nebulised amiloride has been shown to have a small effect in that regard, and newer agents such as adenosine triphosphate (ATP) and uridine triphosphate (UTP) analogues are being assessed. Attempts at modifying the inflammatory response involve the assessment of the role of some currently available (e.g. ibuprofen, azithromycin) and some novel **anti-inflammatory agents** (e.g. pentoxifylline, anti-elastases, serum leucocyte proteinase inhibitors). Improvements in the field of **lung transplantation** offer the best hope for patients in the advanced stages of the disease. Advances in many different areas of scientific research are being brought into clinical practice in order to improve the outlook for patients with cystic fibrosis.

Further reading

Boucher RC. New concepts of the pathogenesis of cystic fibrosis lung disease. *Eur Respir J* 2004; **23**: 146–58.

Cystic Fibrosis Foundation (USA). Website: www.cff.org

Cystic Fibrosis Trust (UK). Website: www.cftrust-org.uk

Davis PB. Cystic fibrosis since 1938. *Am J Respir Crit Care Med* 2006; **173**: 475–82.

Elborn JS, Shale DJ, Britton JR. Cystic fibrosis: current survival and population estimates to the year 2000. *Thorax* 1991; **46**: 881–5.

Elkins MR, Robinson M, Rose BR et al. A controlled trial of long term inhaled hypertonic saline in patients with cystic fibrosis. *N Engl J Med* 2006; **354**: 229–40.

Geddes D. Translational research-from gene to treatment: lessons from cystic fibrosis. *Clin Med* 2005; **5**: 258–63.

Jones AM. Eradication therapy for early *Pseudomonas aeruginosa* infection in CF: many questions still unanswered. *Eur Respir J* 2005; **26**: 373–5.

Price J. Newborn screening for cystic fibrosis. *Arch Dis Child* 2006; **91**: 209–10.

Southern KW, Barker PM. Azithromycin for cystic fibrosis. *Eur Respir J* 2004; **24**: 834–8.

Keypoints

- Cystic fibrosis is a multisystem disease resulting from mutations of a gene which codes for a chloride channel on epithelial membranes.
- In the lungs viscid secretions predispose to infection and inflammation with progressive bronchiectasis.
- *Staphylococcus aureus*, *Pseudomonas aeruginosa* and *Burkholderia cepacia complex* are the main pathogens.
- Antibiotics, chest physiotherapy, nutritional support and anti-inflammatory drugs are key elements in treatment.
- Lung transplantation is the main option to be considered for patients with advanced lung disease.

Chapter 11

Asthma

Definition

Asthma is a disease characterised by **chronic airway inflammation** with **increased airway responsiveness** resulting in **symptoms** such as wheeze, cough and dyspnoea, and **airways obstruction** which is **variable** over short periods of time or **reversible** with treatment.

It is not a static uniform disease state but rather a **dynamic heterogeneous clinical syndrome** which has a number of **different patterns** and which may progress through different stages so that not all features of the disease may be present in an individual patient at a particular point in time. For example, many patients with well-controlled asthma are asymptomatic with normal lung function between attacks although if further investigations were performed there would be evidence of airway inflammation and increased airway responsiveness. By contrast, in some patients with chronic asthma the disease may have progressed to a state of irreversible airways obstruction. Some patients with smoking-related chronic obstructive pulmonary disease (COPD), bronchiectasis or cystic fibrosis may demonstrate airways obstruction with a degree of reversibility but it is important to appreciate that these diseases are different from asthma with distinct aetiologies, pathologies, natural history and responses to treatment.

Prevalence

Asthma has been recognised since ancient times and it is now estimated that 300 million people worldwide have asthma. The term is derived from the Greek word ασθμα, meaning short-drawn breath or panting and was in use in the time of Hippocrates (460–370 BC), although it was probably used to refer to many different causes of breathlessness. This problem of terminology continues in that the reported prevalence of asthma greatly depends on the criteria used to define asthma and is confused by changes in diagnostic habit (**labelling shift**) whereby patients may now be diagnosed as having asthma whereas previously they were labelled as having 'wheezy bronchitis' in the case of children, or 'COPD' in the case of adults, for example. However, despite such labelling shifts there is a general consensus that the **prevalence of asthma is gradually increasing**. Studies using objective measures of reversible airways obstruction and airway hyper-responsiveness in combination with symptoms suggest that **about 7% of the adult population in the UK have asthma**. There is considerable interest in the reasons for the increasing prevalence of asthma and it is likely that such changes relate to environmental rather than genetic factors.

Aetiology (Fig. 11.1)

Asthma is multifactorial in origin, arising from a complex interaction of **genetic** and **environmental** factors. It seems likely that airway inflammation occurs when genetically susceptible individuals are exposed to certain environmental factors but the exact processes underlying asthma may vary from patient to patient. In many cases the most important environmental factors are the intensity, timing and mode of exposure to **aeroallergens** which stimulate the production of IgE. Additional environmental determinants are the concurrent exposure to **cofactors** such as cigarette smoke, atmospheric pollutants and respiratory tract infections.

Genetic susceptibility

There is strong evidence of a hereditary contribution to the aetiology of asthma. It has long been known that asthma and atopy run in **families**. First-degree relatives of asthmatics have a significantly higher prevalence of asthma than relatives of non-asthmatic patients. It is important to appreciate, however, that families share environments

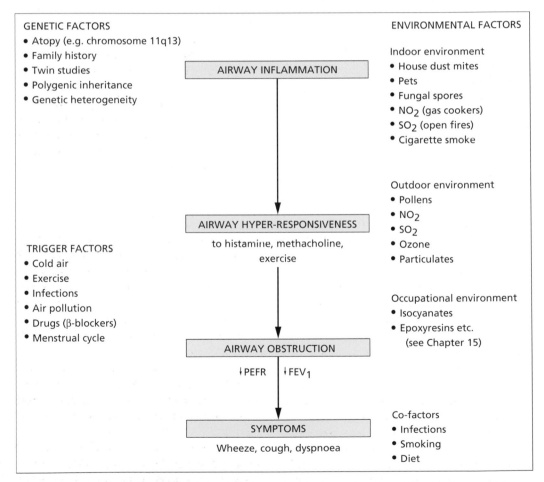

GENETIC FACTORS
- Atopy (e.g. chromosome 11q13)
- Family history
- Twin studies
- Polygenic inheritance
- Genetic heterogeneity

AIRWAY INFLAMMATION

AIRWAY HYPER-RESPONSIVENESS
to histamine, methacholine, exercise

TRIGGER FACTORS
- Cold air
- Exercise
- Infections
- Air pollution
- Drugs (β-blockers)
- Menstrual cycle

AIRWAY OBSTRUCTION
↓PEFR   ↓FEV$_1$

SYMPTOMS
Wheeze, cough, dyspnoea

ENVIRONMENTAL FACTORS

Indoor environment
- House dust mites
- Pets
- Fungal spores
- NO$_2$ (gas cookers)
- SO$_2$ (open fires)
- Cigarette smoke

Outdoor environment
- Pollens
- NO$_2$
- SO$_2$
- Ozone
- Particulates

Occupational environment
- Isocyanates
- Epoxyresins etc. (see Chapter 15)

Co-factors
- Infections
- Smoking
- Diet

Figure 11.1 Asthma is multifactorial in origin, arising from a complex interaction of genetic and environmental factors, which result in airway inflammation and hyper-responsiveness, such that bronchoconstriction develops in response to a variety of trigger factors.

as well as sharing genes, and that environmental factors are necessary for the expression of a genetic predisposition. **Atopy** is a constitutional tendency to produce significant amounts of IgE on exposure to small amounts of common antigens. Atopic individuals demonstrate positive reactions to antigens on skin prick tests and have a high prevalence of asthma, allergic rhinitis, urticaria and eczema. Several potential gene linkages (e.g. chromosome 11q13 location) to asthma and atopy have been suggested but it is clear that the genetic contribution to asthma is complex, possibly involving **polygenic inheritance** (several genes contributing to the asthmatic tendency in an individual) and **genetic heterogeneity** (different combinations of genes causing the asthmatic tendency in different individuals). Recently the ADAM33 gene on chromosome 20p13, which is a disintegrin and metalloprotease gene, has been identified as being involved in the structural airway components of asthma, such as airway remodelling, which relates to the development of chronic persistent asthma with irreversible (fixed) airways obstruction and excess decline in FEV_1 over time.

Environmental factors

The importance of environmental factors in the aetiology of asthma has been particularly evident in studies of populations who have **migrated from one country to another**. For example, children from the Pacific atoll of Tokelau were found to have developed asthma with similar prevalence to native New Zealand children when they were evacuated to New Zealand following a typhoon which devastated the local economy, whereas children remaining in Tokelau had a significantly lesser prevalence. Similarly, movement of people from East to West Germany in the 1990s was associated with an increased incidence of asthma and atopy. It is likely that the increasing prevalence of asthma relates to environmental rather than genetic factors. There may be very many aspects of the environment which are important but a change to a **modern, urban, economically developed society seems to be particularly associated with the occurrence of asthma.**

Indoor environment

People spend at least 75% of their time indoors and overall exposure to air pollutants and allergens is determined more by concentrations indoors than outdoors. The indoor environment is particularly important in the case of young children because allergen exposure early in life may be particularly important in determining sensitisation. There is a vast array of antigens in the typical home environment. **House dust mites** (*Dermatophagoides pteronyssinus*) are found in high concentrations in carpets, soft furnishings and bedding. **Pet-derived allergens** are widespread in homes where dogs, cats or budgerigars are kept. **Feathers** are often present in pillows and duvets. Other antigens commonly present in homes are **fungal spores** and antigens from cockroaches. Pollutants such as **nitrogen dioxide** are commonly found at higher concentrations indoors than outside as a result of sources such as gas cookers and kerosene heaters. **Sulphur dioxide** and **particulate pollutants** are released from open fires or paraffin stoves. Passive exposure to **cigarette smoke** in the home has an adverse effect on asthma and other respiratory diseases in children in particular.

Outdoor environment

Although there is a widespread view among the general public that the increasing prevalence of asthma is attributable to atmospheric pollution from motor vehicles, the balance of evidence suggests that any such influence on the *initiation* of asthma is small. However, outdoor air quality plays an important, although complex and incompletely understood, part in *triggering exacerbations* of pre-existing asthma. Experimental and population studies have shown that nitrogen dioxide, ozone, sulphur dioxide and airborne particulates may have acute adverse effects on asthma during air pollution episodes.

- *Nitrogen dioxide (NO_2)*: the principal source of nitrogen dioxide and other nitrogen oxides (NO_x) is **motor vehicle emissions** but power stations and **fuel-burning industries** also contribute. Nitrogen dioxide is also a common contaminant of indoor air arising from **gas cookers** and kerosene heaters. Nitrogen dioxide reacts with hydrocarbons and oxygen in the presence of sunlight, forming ozone. Emissions of nitrogen dioxide have increased over the last 30 years. Use of catalytic converters in cars reduces exhaust emissions.

• *Sulphur dioxide (SO$_2$)* is created by the **burning of fossil fuels** containing sulphur. **Power stations** are the main source of sulphur dioxide emissions although **domestic coal burning** is an important source in some areas. Diesel vehicles also emit sulphur dioxide. Levels of sulphur dioxide emissions are gradually declining.

• *Ozone (O$_3$)* is formed by a photochemical reaction involving sunlight, oxygen and nitrogen dioxide. Its production is dependent on **weather conditions**. Although nitrogen dioxide and sulphur dioxide levels tend to be higher in cities, ozone levels tend to be higher in rural areas.

• *Airborne particulates*: this is a term used to describe elements of **black smoke** consisting of small particles produced by incomplete combustion.

• *Antigens*: levels of grass and flower **pollens** vary considerably depending on the climatic conditions and time of year, as do levels of **allergens** from rape seed, soy bean and other plants and crops.

Interactions between atmospheric pollutants, aeroallergens and climatic conditions have complex effects on asthma. Some studies suggest that exposure to **air pollution** may enhance airway responses to common **allergens**, thereby potentially having a role in both the initiation of asthma and in the triggering of acute attacks. **Climatic conditions** such as high pressure and humidity with calm still air can result in an accumulation of airborne pollutants (e.g. particulates, ozone) and of allergens (e.g. pollens, fungal spores). Investigation of several epidemics of asthma in Barcelona in the 1980s established that the number of patients referred to hospital with acute attacks of asthma coincided with days when soy bean was being unloaded from ships in the port in conditions of high barometric pressure and little wind. Several epidemics of acute asthma have been associated with thunderstorms, and these have particularly affected patients with pre-existing atopic asthma and IgE reactions to specific antigens such as pollens and fungal spores. Warm dry weather may cause a rapid rise in pollen concentrations and also in levels of O$_3$, nitrogen dioxide and sulphur dioxide because of atmospheric stability. Gusts of wind at the start of a thunderstorm lift allergens into the air. Rain disrupts pollen grains into a number of smaller allergenic particles. Under these circumstances atopic individuals with pre-existing asthma or hay fever are particularly vulnerable to the resultant allergen challenge. The effects of atmospheric pollutants and allergens on asthmatics is influenced by factors such as use of asthma medication, time spent outdoors and exercise (which increases ventilation).

Occupational environment

Many agents encountered in the workplace may induce **occupational asthma** (e.g. isocyanates, epoxyresins, persulphates, hard wood dusts (see Chapter 15)).

Co-factors in asthma

A number of other factors influence the development of asthma.

• *Infections*: many respiratory infections (e.g. influenza A, *Mycoplasma pneumoniae*, *Chlamydia pneumoniae*) provoke a transient increase in airway responsiveness in normal individuals and in asthmatics. Conversely, there is some evidence that viral infections (e.g. measles) in the first year of life may protect against asthma.

• *Smoking*: cigarette **smoking** is associated with increased levels of IgE and with increased sensitisation to certain occupational allergens in particular (e.g. anhydrides). **Maternal smoking** during pregnancy is thought to increase the risk of developing atopic disease in infancy and **passive exposure** to smoking has an adverse effect on asthma and other respiratory diseases.

• *Diet*: some studies suggest that **breast feeding** may offer protection against the subsequent development of asthma, possibly because of reduced exposure to food allergens in the neonatal period. Airway responsiveness may be influenced by dietary **salt intake**, although studies show conflicting results. In some patients asthmatic attacks may occasionally be precipitated by certain foods such as milk, egg, wheat and food **additives** and preservatives (e.g. tartrazine). Diets high in **oily fish** appear to be protective.

- *Drugs*: β-**blocking drugs** can induce bronchoconstriction in asthmatics, sometimes even when given in eye drops (e.g. timolol for glaucoma). A small percentage of asthmatics develop bronchoconstriction when given **salicylates** (e.g. aspirin) or **non-steroidal anti-inflammatory drugs** (e.g. ibuprofen). These drugs block arachidonic acid metabolism down the prostaglandin pathway diverting it to the leukotriene pathway. A reaction to aspirin is more common in asthmatics with nasal polyps.

Pathogenesis and pathology (Fig. 11.2)

A series of factors combine to produce increasing airway inflammation and airway responsiveness, and when these features reach a sufficient level bronchoconstriction and asthma symptoms are triggered. Typically, the inhalation of an allergen in a sensitised atopic asthmatic results in a two-phase response consisting of an **early asthmatic** **reaction** reaching its maximum at about 20 minutes, and a **late asthmatic reaction** developing about 6–12 hours later. These atopic asthmatics have high levels of specific IgE which binds to receptors on inflammatory cells, most notably mast cells. Interaction of the IgE antibody and inhaled antigen results in the activation of these inflammatory cells and release of preformed mediators such as histamine, prostaglandins and leukotrienes which cause contraction of smooth muscle of the airways producing bronchoconstriction. The inflammatory response in asthma is highly complex involving the full **spectrum of inflammatory cells** including mast cells, eosinophils, B and T lymphocytes and neutrophils, which release an **array of mediators and cytokines**. These mediators regulate the response of other inflammatory cells, and have a number of effects resulting in **contraction of airway smooth muscle, increased vascular permeability** and stimulation of airway **mucus secretion**. T-helper lymphocytes have an important role in the regulation of the inflammatory response. These cells may be divided into two main subsets on the basis of the profile of cytokines which they produce. **Th2 cells** produce interleukin 4 (IL-4), IL-5, IL-6 and IL-10 and **up-regulate** the specific form of airway inflammation of asthma

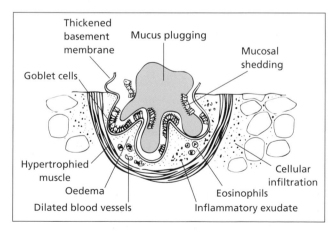

Figure 11.2 The pathogenesis and pathology of asthma. Asthma is characterised by a complex pattern of airway inflammation as a result of an interaction of genetic and environmental factors. Eosinophils, mast cells, neutrophils, B and T cells are all involved in the cellular infiltration. Mediators and cytokines regulate the inflammatory response and result in contraction of airway smooth muscle, increased permeability of blood vessels and mucus secretion. In chronic asthma airway remodelling results in structural changes and fixed airways obstruction.

by enhancing IgE synthesis and eosinophil and mast-cell function. In contrast, **Th1 cells** produce IL-2, interferon γ (IFN-γ) and lymphotoxin and **down-regulate the atopic response**. In those who are genetically susceptible to developing asthma, antigen presentation to T-helper cells leads to a Th2 response. Infection with respiratory syncytial virus augments a Th2 response, whereas some other microbial antigens lead to a Th1 response. It has been suggested that exposure to allergens and infections in early childhood is important in determining the pattern of immune response thereby modulating the genetic susceptibility to developing asthma. In affluent countries declining family size, improved household amenities and higher standards of cleanliness seem to be associated with an increased incidence of asthma. The **'hygiene hypothesis'** suggests that allergic diseases may be prevented by certain infections in early childhood. Thus, for example, children with older siblings are more likely to be exposed to childhood infections and have a lower incidence of asthma.

The wall of the airway in asthma is thickened by oedema, cellular infiltration, increased smooth-muscle mass and glands (Fig. 11.2). With increasing severity and chronicity of the disease **remodelling of the airway** occurs leading to fibrosis of the airway wall, fixed narrowing of the airway and a reduced response to bronchodilator medication. Mucus plugging of the lumen of the airway is a prominent feature of acute severe asthma. Although in clinical practice patients with asthma are sometimes classified as having atopic asthma (occurring in relation to inhalation of environmental antigens in a susceptible person) or non-atopic asthma (occurring without any definable relationship to an environmental antigen), the pathological features of the airway inflammation are identical. It is likely that the inflammatory cascade of asthma can be initiated by a variety of different factors in different patients.

Clinical features

The typical symptoms of asthma are **wheeze, dyspnoea, cough** and a sensation of **'chest tightness'**. These symptoms may occur for the first time at any age and may be episodic or persistent. In **episodic asthma** the patient is often asymptomatic between episodes but suffers attacks of asthma during viral respiratory tract infections or after exposure to certain allergens. This pattern of asthma is commonly seen in children and young adults who have IgE antibodies to common inhaled antigens (e.g. grass pollens, pet dander), and the term **'atopic asthma'** is used. Sometimes the clinical pattern is of **persistent asthma** with chronic wheeze and dyspnoea. This pattern is more common in older patients with **'adult-onset'** asthma who are non-atopic and whose symptoms are not related to any apparent antigen exposure so that the term **'non-atopic asthma'** is sometimes used. The variable nature of symptoms is a characteristic feature of asthma. Typically, there is a diurnal pattern with symptoms and peak expiratory flow measurements being worse early in the morning—so-called **'morning dipping'**. Symptoms such as cough and wheeze often disturb sleep and the term **'nocturnal asthma'** emphasises this. Cough is often the dominant symptom and the lack of wheeze or dyspnoea may lead to a delay in making the diagnosis: so-called, **'cough variant asthma'**. Symptoms may be provoked by exercise: **'exercise asthma'**. These descriptive clinical terms are useful in emphasising some characteristic features of asthma, and highlight the fact that asthma is not a uniform static disease but a broad dynamic clinical syndrome.

When assessing a patient with confirmed or suspected asthma it is important to focus on key aspects of the history which not only aid diagnosis but which are also important in assessing the pattern of the asthma and in treatment.

- *Family history*: there is a significantly increased prevalence of asthma in relatives of patients with asthma or other atopic diseases (eczema, hay fever, allergic rhinitis).
- *Home environment*: smoking, or exposure to passive smoking in the home environment, is an adverse factor. Indoor allergens, for example house dust mite, dog or cat dander may be important in triggering attacks.
- *Occupational history*: it is important to identify if the patient's asthma could have been caused by

exposure to asthmagenic agents at work, by enquiring about current and previous jobs, the tasks performed and materials used. Do symptoms improve away from work at weekends or on holidays? Are symptoms worse on return to work, particularly the evening or night after work (see Chapter 15)?

- *Trigger factors*: are there any factors which precipitate symptoms?

(a) Exercise

(b) Cold air

(c) Viral respiratory infections

(d) Allergen exposure (e.g. feather pillows, cat dander)

(e) Seasonal factors (e.g. grass pollen)

(f) Drugs (e.g. β-blockers, aspirin)

- *Response to treatment*: enquiry about the effectiveness of previous treatment with bronchodilator drugs or prednisolone yields clues to the reversibility of the disease and is particularly important in detecting asthma in older patients who may have been erroneously labelled as having COPD.

The characteristic features on examination of patients with asthma are diffuse bilateral **wheeze** (rhonchi) and a **prolonged expiratory phase** to respiration, but there are often no signs detectable between episodes. There may be features of associated diseases such as allergic rhinitis, nasal polyps and eczema. It is essential to be alert for atypical features such as unilateral wheeze which suggests local bronchial obstruction by a foreign body (e.g. inhaled peanut) in a child or a carcinoma in an adult, for example. It is also important to ensure that there are no signs of cardiac or other respiratory disease. During acute attacks of asthma features such as tachycardia, tachypnoea, cyanosis, use of accessory muscles of respiration and features of anxiety and general distress indicate a severe episode. Pulsus paradoxus (a fall of more than 10 mmHg in systolic blood pressure during inspiration) may be present but is an unreliable indicator of severity. Chronic severe childhood asthma may cause chest deformity with the sternum being pushed forwards (pigeon chest deformity) and the lower rib cage being pulled inwards (Harrison's sulcus) but these features are rarely seen nowadays.

Investigations

Lung function tests

The key feature of asthma is airways obstruction which is variable over short periods of time or reversible with treatment. Measurement of airways obstruction using a peak expiratory flow meter or spirometer is as essential in assessing a patient with asthma as measurement of blood pressure using a sphygmomanometer is in a patient with hypertension.

- *Airways obstruction*: peak expiratory flow, forced expiratory volume in 1 second (FEV_1) and FEV_1/ vital capacity (VC) ratio are reduced in active asthma. However, asthma is a dynamic condition and peak expiratory flow rate (PEFR) and spirometry may be normal between attacks in a patient with episodic asthma.

- *Reversibility*: if airways obstruction is detected by peak flow or spirometry the next step is to assess its reversibility to **bronchodilator drugs**. Typically, the patient is given 200 μg salbutamol and spirometry or peak flow measurements are repeated 15–20 minutes later. Patients with active asthma characteristically show airways obstruction with a large bronchodilator response ($FEV_1 > 15\%$ improvement and at least 200 mL; PEFR $> 20\%$ improvements and at least 60 L/min). Patients with more severe chronic asthma may fail to show an improvement after a bronchodilator drug but demonstrate reversibility to **steroids**. A therapeutic trial of prednisolone 30 mg/day for 14 days often results in a marked improvement in airways obstruction in patients who have failed to show reversibility to bronchodilator drugs.

- *Variability:* the variability of the airways obstruction of asthma is demonstrated by **serial measurements of peak flow** or spirometry over a period of time. The patient is given a peak flow meter and taught to record measurements. A characteristic pattern is '**morning dipping**' in which peak flow values are lowest in the morning, improving throughout the day. This diurnal variability is most marked in active, poorly controlled asthma. A 20% or greater variability in amplitude % best

PEFR (i.e. highest − lowest/highest × 100) with a minimum change of 60 L/min is highly suggestive of asthma. Serial peak flow measurements may also be used to demonstrate the variability of airways obstruction in relation to factors such as exercise or environmental allergens, for example.

Total lung capacity is usually increased in asthma as a manifestation of **hyperinflation**, and residual volume is elevated indicating **air trapping**. In contrast to patients with COPD (see Chapter 12), the airways obstruction of asthma is not associated with any impairment of gas diffusion so that transfer factor for carbon monoxide ($T_L\text{CO}$) and transfer coefficient ($K\text{CO}$) are characteristically normal or indeed slightly elevated. During an acute severe attack of asthma, **hypoxaemia** develops and is usually associated with increased ventilation and a reduced $P\text{CO}_2$. Elevation of $P\text{CO}_2$ in a patient with asthma is a sign of a critically ill patient who is failing to maintain ventilation.

Airway responsiveness

Airway responsiveness is a measure of the general **'irritability' of the airways**, the degree to which **bronchoconstriction develops in response to physical or chemical stimuli**.

- *Exercise testing*: one of the most useful ways of demonstrating increased airway responsiveness or hyper-reactivity is to measure peak flow or spirometry before and after 5–10 minutes of vigorous exercise. A post-exercise fall in FEV_1 or peak flow of 20%

is highly suggestive of asthma, as normal subjects usually show a degree of bronchodilatation, rather than bronchoconstriction, during exercise. An **exercise provocation test** is most useful if a patient with suspected asthma has normal peak flow or spirometry when seen in the clinic, such that reversibility testing may be of little use, and a 'provocation' test is more useful. The response is greater if exercise is performed in cold air.

- *Histamine/methacholine provocation tests*: the degree of airway responsiveness can be measured precisely in the laboratory. Under careful supervision the patient inhales increasing doses of nebulised **histamine** or **methacholine**, starting at a very low dose, and serial spirometry is performed. By plotting the percentage fall in FEV_1 the concentration (C), or dose (D), of the chemical provoking (P) a 20% fall in FEV_1, can be calculated and expressed as a figure (e.g. PD_{20} methacholine 200 μg or PC_{20} histamine 4 mg/mL). Histamine or methacholine provocation tests are not usually required for the diagnosis of asthma in routine practice but are particularly useful in assessing changes in airway responsiveness in relation to exposure to environmental or occupational allergens (see Chapter 15), and in research studies.

Tests for hypersensitivity

Skin prick tests (Fig. 11.3) may be performed to identify atopy and to detect particular sensitivity to a specific antigen with a view to exclusion of

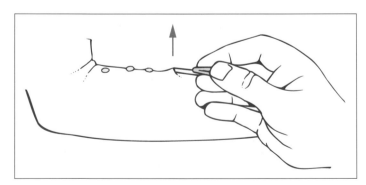

Figure 11.3 Skin prick test. Drops of antigen extracts and antigen-free control solution are placed on the flexor surface of the forearm. Each drop is pricked with a fine needle. The needle is held parallel to the skin surface, advanced slightly and a tiny fold of skin lifted briefly as shown. Deep stabs and bleeding should be avoided. Weal and flare are measured after 10–20 minutes.

exposure where possible (e.g. cat allergens). Drops of antigen extracts are placed on the flexor surface of the forearm and the tip of a small stylet is pressed into the superficial epidermis through the drop of allergen. A positive reaction is manifest as a weal with a surrounding erythematous flare at about 15 minutes. The reaction to allergens should be compared with the reaction to a drop of histamine and to a drop of control solution containing no antigens. Total **IgE level** is often elevated in patients with atopic asthma and they sometimes have a mild peripheral blood **eosinophilia. Radioallergosorbent testing (RAST)** is a means of measuring the level of circulating IgE specifically directed towards a particular antigen.

Some asthmatics develop an allergic reaction to *Aspergillus fumigatus*, a ubiquitous fungus which may colonise the airways. In these circumstances the asthma is typically severe and persistent requiring systemic steroid treatment. There is often associated severe airway inflammation and mucus plugging resulting in bronchiectasis (see Chapter 9). In addition to a positive skin prick test to *Aspergillus* these patients often have significant eosinophilia and **precipitating antibodies to *Aspergillus*** in their serum. Very rarely, asthma occurs as part of an eosinophilic vasculitis such as Churg–Strauss syndrome (see Chapter 16), in which case very high levels of blood eosinophilia occur.

General investigations

Further general investigations may be necessary to exclude other cardiorespiratory diseases. **Chest X-ray** is essential in older patients who have smoked, to exclude bronchial carcinoma, for example, and may be needed in children if there are any clinical features to suggest other diseases such as cystic fibrosis or bronchiectasis. **Bronchoscopy** is occasionally necessary to assess for vocal cord dysfunction, inhaled foreign bodies, bronchial carcinoma or rarer causes of bronchial obstruction such as carcinoid tumours. **Exhaled nitric oxide** (NO) levels are increased in patients with asthma and this is a marker of airway inflammation which can be measured non-invasively. The equipment needed to measure exhaled NO is expensive and this test is mainly used in research studies rather than in routine clinical practice.

Diagnosis (Table 11.1)

Although diagnosing asthma is straightforward when the patient presents with classic symptoms and evidence of variable or reversible airways obstruction, there are many pitfalls, and errors in diagnosis are common. **Failure to diagnose** asthma results in the patient being deprived of appropriate asthma treatment, for example a child with cough receiving recurrent courses of antibiotics for 'chest infections' when in fact he or she is suffering from asthma. Conversely, **incorrect diagnosis** of asthma might expose the patient to the risks of inappropriate treatment (e.g. recurrent courses of prednisolone) and delay appropriate management of other lung disease, e.g. inhaled foreign body in a child or tracheal tumour in an adult producing **wheeze simulating asthma**. On the one hand it

Table 11.1 Diagnosing asthma. 'All that wheezes is not asthma and not all asthma wheezes'.

Underdiagnosis: Could this patient's symptoms be caused by asthma?
Overdiagnosis: Does this patient really have asthma?
• Recognise **symptoms** suggestive of asthma (e.g. wheeze, cough, recurrent 'chest infections')
• Establish evidence of **airways obstruction** (e.g. ↓ peak flow, ↓ FEV_1, ↓ FEV_1/VC ratio)
• Assess **variability**, **reversibility**, **provocability** of airway obstruction: serial peak flow chart (e.g. morning dipping; response to bronchodilator and steroid trial; exercise-induced fall in peak flow)
• **Monitor** progress and **review diagnosis** (e.g. has 'wheezy bronchitis' of childhood evolved into established asthma or was it a result of viral bronchiolitis?)
• Consider **additional diagnoses** (e.g. occupational asthma, allergic bronchopulmonary aspergillosis)
• Exclude alternative diagnoses (e.g. cystic fibrosis, COPD, carcinoma, inhaled foreign body)

COPD, chronic obstructive pulmonary disease; FEV_1, forced expiratory volume in 1 second; VC, vital capacity.

is necessary to be alert to less well-recognised presentations of asthma, for example cough without wheeze, and on the other hand to be prepared to review the evidence for asthma if the response to treatment is poor or if unusual features emerge (e.g. could this child possibly have cystic fibrosis?). Evidence establishing the diagnosis of asthma and excluding other diseases often emerges over time and it is sometimes wise to use interim terms such as **'suspected asthma'** while gathering evidence of variable or reversible airways obstruction that allows a **firm diagnosis** of asthma to be established. Doubt may arise where it is difficult to obtain accurate peak flow or spirometry measurements as in the case of young children. Even when the diagnosis of asthma is established the diagnostic process should be taken further: **could this be occupational asthma?** Is there evidence of additional lung disease such as bronchiectasis or allergic bronchopulmonary aspergillosis? The doctor needs to exercise good clinical skills in applying two critical questions: **could this patient's symptoms be caused by asthma? Does this patient really have asthma?**

Management (Fig. 11.4)

Patient education

Successful management of asthma requires that **patients**, or the **parents** of a child with asthma, understand the nature of the condition and its treatment. Patient education should begin at the time of diagnosis and form part of every subsequent consultation between the patient and **doctor**. All members of the **team** should participate in the process and there is a particular role for respiratory **nurse specialists**.

Education involves the patient understanding the **nature of asthma**, learning the **practical skills** necessary to manage asthma and adopting the appropriate actions in managing their asthma and **using their medication**. Education of the patient often starts with a discussion of the multifactorial aetiology of asthma and identification of **precipitating factors**. It is useful for patients to understand that inflammation of the airways is a key factor underlying the development of wheeze as they can then

appreciate the difference between **'reliever'** (bronchodilator) and **'preventer'** (anti-inflammatory) medication. Sufficient time should be invested in instructing the patient in the **use of inhaler devices**, as this is a crucial aspect determining the effectiveness of prescribed medication.

Use of a **peak flow meter** provides patients with an objective measure of airway obstruction allowing them to see the variability of readings from day to day, the influence of precipitating factors and the effect of treatment. Most patients with asthma should be able to **monitor and manage** their asthma themselves to a considerable degree and to recognise when medical advice is needed, in much the same way as patients with diabetes monitor their blood sugar levels and adjust insulin therapy.

The amount of information given to each patient needs to be varied in accordance with their needs and aptitude but all patients should know about features which indicate when their asthma is deteriorating and what action to take in these circumstances. Healthcare professionals should be aware that it is often those patients least interested in learning about their disease who are at greatest risk and that features such as depression, anxiety, denial of disease and non-adherence with treatment are strongly associated with asthma deaths. Particular effort is required to identify and target resources at such patients. Information conveyed in discussion with the patient should be supplemented by **personalised written information**. Many patients are frightened and anxious about the diagnosis of asthma and it is often helpful to point out that many top-class sports men and women have asthma which does not impair their performance. Many such sports people lend their support to organisations such as the National Asthma Campaign in the UK which provide literature and support to help patients with asthma.

Avoidance of precipitating factors

Most patients with atopic asthma react to many different antigens so that environmental control measures are generally not particularly helpful. **House dust mites** are most prevalent in warm moist areas

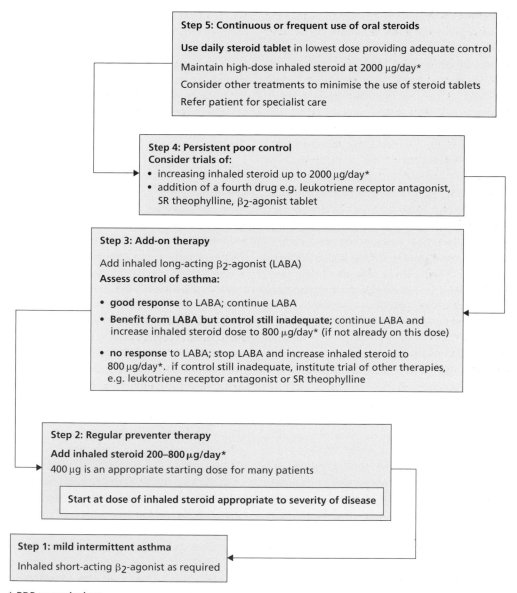

Step 5: Continuous or frequent use of oral steroids

Use daily steroid tablet in lowest dose providing adequate control

Maintain high-dose inhaled steroid at 2000 μg/day*

Consider other treatments to minimise the use of steroid tablets

Refer patient for specialist care

Step 4: Persistent poor control
Consider trials of:
- increasing inhaled steroid up to 2000 μg/day*
- addition of a fourth drug e.g. leukotriene receptor antagonist, SR theophylline, β₂-agonist tablet

Step 3: Add-on therapy

Add inhaled long-acting β₂-agonist (LABA)
Assess control of asthma:

- **good response** to LABA; continue LABA
- **Benefit form LABA but control still inadequate;** continue LABA and increase inhaled steroid dose to 800 μg/day* (if not already on this dose)
- **no response** to LABA; stop LABA and increase inhaled steroid to 800 μg/day*. if control still inadequate, institute trial of other therapies, e.g. leukotriene receptor antagonist or SR theophylline

Step 2: Regular preventer therapy

Add inhaled steroid 200–800 μg/day*
400 μg is an appropriate starting dose for many patients

Start at dose of inhaled steroid appropriate to severity of disease

Step 1: mild intermittent asthma

Inhaled short-acting β₂-agonist as required

* **BDP or equivalent**

Figure 11.4 Summary of the stepwise management of asthma in adults (Reproduced with permission from British Thoracic Society/Scottish Intercollegiate Guidelines Network British guideline on the management of asthma – 2005 (http//www.brit-thoracic.org.uk)).

containing desquamated human skin scales and they are almost universally distributed in mattresses, pillows, carpets, furnishings and soft toys. The level of house dust mite can be reduced by encasing mattresses in occlusive covers and by frequent washing of blankets and duvets. Humidity levels can be decreased by better ventilation. Avoidance of exposure to **pet allergens** from dogs or cats, for example, is more feasible but the result of these interventions is often disappointing. Similarly, it is difficult to avoid exposure to **outdoor allergens** but some patients benefit from precautions such as increasing asthma treatment or remaining indoors with closed windows when pollen counts are high.

Desensitisation (immunotherapy) is a highly specialised technique in which repeated injections of an allergen are given to a sensitised subject in an attempt to produce 'blocking antibody' of IgG type which prevents the allergen binding to specific IgE on mast cells. It is most commonly used in the treatment of well-documented life-threatening anaphylactic reactions to insect stings but there is little evidence of its benefit in asthma and there are major concerns about the risk of anaphylaxis.

Avoidance of irritants such as **cigarette smoke** or generally dusty environments is advisable. **Avoidance of** β-blocker drugs is important for all patients with asthma, and patients who are sensitive to **aspirin** should avoid all aspirin-containing products and non-steroidal anti-inflammatory drugs. **Viral infections** often precipitate attacks of asthma so that it is advisable for patients to monitor peak flow measurements carefully during such infections and to intensify asthma treatment as required. Because influenza infection may precipitate severe exacerbations of asthma, annual **influenza vaccination** is recommended.

Exercise is a particular factor precipitating asthma. Bronchoconstriction may develop within minutes of onset of vigorous activity. This response usually resolves within 30 minutes and there then follows a refractory period of about 2 hours when further exercise does not provoke bronchoconstriction. Therefore a warm-up period before the main exercise usually controls this problem. Use of β-agonist medication or sodium cromoglycate before exercise often prevents exercise-induced asthma, allowing athletes with asthma to compete at the highest level of their sport. For example, 67 athletes at the 1984 Olympic Games had asthma, and many won medals!

Drug treatment

Bronchodilator drugs ('relievers') are used to relieve symptoms of bronchoconstriction. **Anti-inflammatory drugs** ('preventers') treat the underlying chronic inflammatory process in asthma. Short courses of oral **prednisolone** ('rescue medication')** are used to treat exacerbations. Most patients with chronic asthma can be managed very satisfactorily with regular inhaled steroids to control airway inflammation, an inhaled bronchodilator to be taken as required to reverse wheezing, and training to initiate emergency prednisolone treatment when needed.

Bronchodilators

- *β2-agonists*: (e.g. salbutamol, terbutaline) stimulate β-adrenoceptors in the smooth muscle of the airway, producing smooth-muscle relaxation and **bronchodilatation**. They have an onset of action within 15 minutes and a duration of action of 4–6 hours. Side-effects include tremor, palpitations and muscle cramps but these are uncommon unless high doses are used. The main concern about bronchodilator medication is that over-reliance on these drugs may disguise the severity of the asthma by providing symptom relief but not control of the underlying inflammatory process (in much the same way as a pain-killer relieves pain but does not treat the cause). Increasing need for bronchodilator medication is an indication of poorly controlled asthma and a need to increase anti-inflammatory medication.

- *Long-acting β2-agonists*: (e.g. salmeterol, formoterol) have a duration of action of more than 12 hours and are particularly helpful in controlling chronic asthma and in improving nocturnal symptoms. Their use is only recommended as an adjunct to inhaled corticosteroids so that control of the airway inflammation is not neglected. Studies have shown a higher incidence of asthma-related adverse events in patients taking a long-acting β2-agonist without inhaled corticosteroids. **Combination inhalers**, which combine a long-acting β2-agonist and a corticosteroid, may be useful in that regard.

- *Anti-muscarinic bronchodilators*: (e.g. ipratropium) produce bronchodilatation by **blocking the bronchoconstrictor effect of vagal nerve** stimulation on bronchial smooth muscle. They take about 1 hour to reach their maximum effect and have a duration of action of about 4–6 hours. Side-effects are uncommon but nebulised anti-cholinergic drugs may be deposited in the eyes, aggravating glaucoma. In most patients with asthma they are less effective than β_2-agonists but they may be useful in young children and older patients.

- *Theophyllines* increase cyclic adenosine monophosphate (cAMP) stimulation of β-adrenoceptors by **inhibiting the metabolism of cAMP** by the enzyme phosphodiesterase. They may also have other effects including some anti-inflammatory actions. They are not available in inhaler form and absorption from the gastrointestinal tract and clearance of the drug by the liver are variable so that the dose needs to be titrated carefully in accordance with blood levels. Side-effects such as nausea, vomiting, headache, tachycardia and malaise are common. Hepatic clearance of theophyllines is reduced by drugs such as cimetidine, ciprofloxacin and erythromycin, and toxicity can occur if these medications are prescribed without adjustment in the dose of theophylline. Aminophylline is an intravenous form of theophylline (combined with ethylenediamine for solubility) which may be used in severe attacks of asthma not responding to β-agonist medication. It must be given slowly (over at least 20 minutes) with careful adjustment of dose in accordance with blood levels in order to avoid serious toxicity such as convulsions and cardiac arrhythmias. It does not usually result in any additional bronchodilatation compared to standard treatment with nebulised bronchodilators and systemic steroids, and side-effects are common so that its use is usually reserved for very severe asthma not responding to standard treatment.
- *Magnesium*: magnesium sulphate (1.2–2 g as an intravenous infusion over 20 minutes) acts as a smooth-muscle relaxant and is safe and effective in treating patients with acute severe asthma who have not had a satisfactory initial response to nebulised salbutamol.

Anti-inflammatory drugs

- *Inhaled corticosteroids* (e.g. beclometasone, budesonide, fluticasone, mometasone, ciclesonide) are the mainstay of asthma treatment because they **counteract airway inflammation** which is the key underlying process in asthma. It is essential that the patient understands that this is a **preventative treatment** which needs to be taken regularly and which does not provide immediate relief of symptoms. **Adherence** is improved by using a twice-daily regimen whereby the patient's 'preventative' steroid inhaler is left at their bedside and taken regularly every night and morning whereas their 'reliever' bronchodilator is carried around with them for use as required. The dose is adjusted to give optimal control and varies greatly from patient to patient. Many adult patients with relatively mild asthma achieve good control with a dosage of about 400 μg/day beclometasone, but some patients with chronic severe asthma may require 2000 μg/day. In adult patients **'low-dose'** (below the equivalent of about 800 μg/day beclometasone) inhaled steroids are not usually associated with any significant adverse effects apart from oropharyngeal candidiasis or hoarseness of the voice which can be reduced by using a spacer device and gargling the throat with water after inhalation. With **'high dose'** inhaled steroids (above about 800 μg/day beclometasone) biochemical evidence of suppression of adrenal function, and increased bone turnover are detectable in some patients. The clinical significance of such systemic effects needs to be considered in the context of the dangers of uncontrolled asthma and alternative therapies such as oral prednisolone. The dosage of inhaled steroids should be reviewed regularly to ensure that the patient is taking as much as is required to control their asthma ('step up') but, equally, as little as necessary ('step down') so as to minimise the risk of adverse effects with long-term usage. Patients taking high dose inhaled corticosteroid should carry a steroid treatment card advising of the risk of adrenal suppression.
- *Sodium cromoglycate* is a preventative inhaled treatment which has a number of anti-inflammatory actions including stabilisation of mast cells. It is mainly used in children with mild asthma and it has no significant adverse effects. However, it is less effective than inhaled steroids in more troublesome asthma. Nedocromil is a newer inhaled compound with similar properties to cromoglycate.
- *Oral steroid treatment*: **'rescue' courses** of oral steroids may be needed to control exacerbations of

asthma. Typically, this consists of 30–40 mg/day prednisolone for about 7–14 days in an adult. Treatment is continued until asthma control has been achieved. Most patients should be taught to start their own short course of oral prednisolone in accordance with a predetermined action plan (e.g. when peak flow falls below 60% of the patient's best value). Patients should understand the potential adverse effects of long-term use of prednisolone and the difference between this and infrequent short-course usage which is safe. A very small number of patients require **long-term systemic prednisolone** to control severe asthma. These patients should be attending a hospital specialist and it should have been clearly established that their asthma cannot be controlled by other measures. The dosage of steroids needs to be kept as low as possible. In these circumstances the patient should be given a **'steroid treatment card'** documenting the dosage of steroids used, advising about adverse effects and warning patients that steroids should not be stopped suddenly because of the risk of adrenal insufficiency. Booster doses may be required during illnesses and patients may be particularly susceptible to infections such as chickenpox: other **adverse effects** include peptic ulceration, myopathy, osteoporosis, growth suppression, depression, psychosis, cataracts and cushingoid features. Patients receiving long-term oral prednisolone should be considered for preventative treatment of osteoporosis such as smoking cessation, exercise, hormone replacement therapy, adequate dietary calcium intake and disodium etidronate/calcium treatment where appropriate.

• *Leukotriene receptor antagonists* (e.g. montelukast, zafirlukast) block the effects of cysteinyl leukotrienes which are metabolites of arachidonic acid with bronchoconstrictor and pro-inflammatory actions. Leukotriene antagonists are a new modality of anti-inflammatory therapy in asthma, which are given orally in tablet form. They improve lung function and reduce bronchial hyper-responsiveness in patients with asthma. These effects are similar to those seen with 400 μg/day beclometasone. Most studies of leukotriene antagonists have shown benefit in patients with mild asthma but

they may also be used as 'add-on' therapy in patients whose asthma is not controlled on inhaled corticosteroids.

• *Anti-IgE treatment* (Omalizumab) is a monoclonal antibody which binds to IgE. It is a new form of add-on therapy for some patients with severe persistent IgE-mediated asthma to inhaled allergens, who are not controlled by high dose inhaled corticosteroid and long-acting β agonist medication. It is administered by subcutaneous injection every 2–4 weeks and the dose depends on the baseline IgE level. Its use is currently restricted to hospital-based physicians who are experienced in the treatment of severe persistent asthma.

Stepwise approach to treatment of asthma (Fig 11.4)

The British Thoracic Society guidelines on the management of asthma recommend a stepwise approach to treatment according to the severity of the asthma in order to gain control of the disease. The aims of treatment are to abolish symptoms, to restore normal or best possible airway function and to reduce the risk of severe attacks as much as possible. Patients should start treatment at the step most appropriate to the initial severity of their asthma and treatment is adjusted as appropriate thereafter. For the majority of patients, asthma is controlled by a combination of a regular inhaled steroid and use of an inhaled bronchodilator drug as required. Bronchodilator drugs are primarily intended to provide symptom relief whereas inhaled steroids are targeted at the underlying inflammatory process in the airways. Treatment should be **'stepped up' as much as necessary** to control the asthma; when control has been achieved treatment may be **'stepped down'** so that the patient is on **no more treatment than is necessary**.

Asthma is a dynamic condition changing over time and ongoing management requires an assessment of the level of control of the asthma that has been achieved and adjustment of medication to find the optimal balance between control of the asthma, use of medication and potential adverse effects of treatment. **Assessing asthma control** involves:

- measurement of peak flow or spirometry and comparing the values with the patient's best value and predicted normal value
- monitoring of serial peak flow records over several days to assess diurnal and day-to-day variability
- assessment of the patient's requirements for use of bronchodilator 'reliever' medication and 'rescue' courses of oral steroids
- noting absences from work or school because of asthma
- assessment of level of symptoms (e.g. nocturnal sleep disturbance or exercise-induced bronchospasm).

Inhaler devices

The inhaled route is preferred for bronchodilator and corticosteroid drugs because it allows these drugs to be delivered directly to the airway reducing the risk of systemic adverse effects. A large number of different inhaler devices and drug formulations are available (Table 11.2). Current evidence suggests that there is no major difference in the clinical effectiveness of the various devices provided the patients is able to use the device appropriately.

- *Metered-dose inhalers* (Fig. 11.5): pressurised metered-dose inhalers were first introduced in 1956 and used chlorofluorocarbons (CFCs) as a propellant. Because of the damaging effect of CFCs to the ozone, CFC inhalers have been phased out over recent years and modern metered-dose inhalers use hydrofluoroalkane (HFA) as a propellant. It is essential to instruct the patient in the correct use of the inhaler (Fig. 11.5) and this should be rechecked frequently. About 10% of the drug is delivered to the lower airways and the remainder is mainly deposited in the oropharynx and swallowed into the gastrointestinal tract where it is absorbed into the blood, but mostly metabolised by first-pass metabolism in the liver.
- *Spacer devices* (e.g. Volumatic®, Nebuhaler®, Aerochamber®) (Fig. 11.6): poor inhaler technique is a significant problem in the use of metered-dose inhalers. Large-volume spacer devices overcome some of these problems and improve deposition of the drugs in the lower airway to about 20% on average. The canister (cr) of pressurised aerosol is inserted into one end of the spacer device and the patient

Table 11.2 Some commonly used inhaler devices and drug formulations in the UK. A large number of different inhaler devices and drug formulations are available. The choice of an inhaler device is based on the patient's preference, the patient's ability to learn to use the device, and the cost and range of medications available in the device.

	β_2-agonist (short-acting)	β_2-agonist (long-acting)	Steroid	Antimuscarinic (short-acting)	Antimuscarinic (long-acting)	Combination Long acting β_2/Steroid	Combination β_2-agonist (short-acting) and anti-cholinergic (short-acting)
Metered Dose Inhaler	√	√	√	√	X	√	√
Autohaler®	√	X	√	X	X	X	X
Easibreathe®	√	X	√	X	X	X	X
Turbohaler®	√	√	√	X	X	√	X
Diskhaler®	√	√	√	X	X	X	X
Accuhaler®	√	√	√	X	X	√	X
Handihaler®	X	X	X	X	√	X	X
Clickhaler®	√	X	√	X	X	X	X

√ – Available; X – Not available.

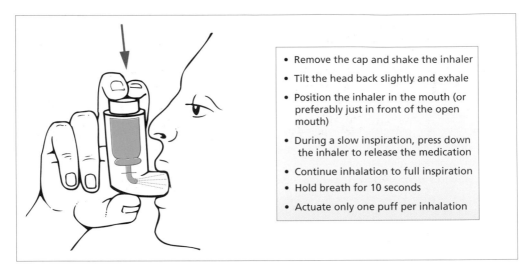

- Remove the cap and shake the inhaler
- Tilt the head back slightly and exhale
- Position the inhaler in the mouth (or preferably just in front of the open mouth)
- During a slow inspiration, press down the inhaler to release the medication
- Continue inhalation to full inspiration
- Hold breath for 10 seconds
- Actuate only one puff per inhalation

Figure 11.5 Pressurised metered-dose inhaler.

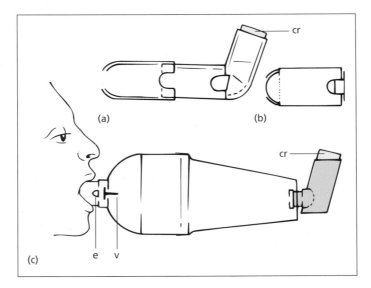

Figure 11.6 Examples of spacer devices for use with metered-dose inhalers. (a) The Spacer-inhaler® is convenient and collapsible (b) and allows the patient to inhale after discharge of the aerosol; (c) the Nebuhaler® (AstraZeneca) is a large-volumed device, designed to allow even freer dispersal of the discharged material so that a high proportion of it forms particles small enough to be inhaled. It also allows large doses of aerosol to be inhaled relatively efficiently (see text). cr: canister of pressurised aerosol, e: expiratory port, v: valve which closes on expiration.

breathes through the other end via a one-way valve (v) which closes on expiration; (e) expiratory port. This **reduces the need for coordination of inspiration and actuation of the inhaler**. Distancing the inhaler from the mouth ('spacing') results in a fine aerosol of smaller particles **improving delivery of** **the drug to the lower airways**. Spacer devices should be cleaned monthly by washing in detergent and allowing them dry in air. They should be replaced at least every 12 months.

- *Breath-actuated aerosol inhalers* (e.g. Autohaler®, Easibreathe®) avoid the need for the patient

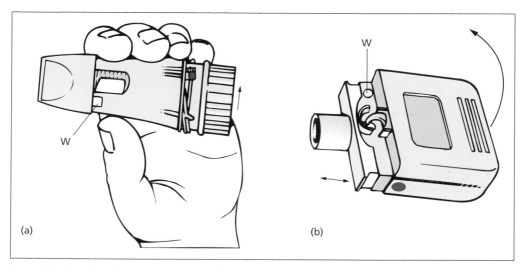

Figure 11.7 Examples of dry-powder inhalers: (a) Turbohaler® (AstraZeneca); (b) Diskhaler (Allen and Hanbury). (a) Turbohaler®: the inhaler is shown with the cover removed, the mouthpiece is to the left. Up to 200 doses of the powdered drug are stored in a reservoir through which the air channel passes. A dose of the dry powder is rotated into the air channel by turning the distal section (arrow). The number of doses remaining is indicated in a small window (w). (b) Diskhaler®: the inhaler is shown with the mouthpiece cover removed; the mouthpiece is to the left. The individual doses are contained in sealed 'blebs' on a disc which is placed on a 'carousel' assembly inside the inhaler. With an in–out movement of the front end of the inhaler (double arrow) the disc rotates and a new bleb moves into place. The bleb is perforated before inhalation by opening the top flap (arrow). When the patient inspires, air is directed through the pierced bleb and the powder is dispersed into the airstream.

to co-ordinate actuation of the inhaler and breathing. The valve on the inhaler is actuated as the patient breathes in, delivering the drug only during inspiration.

• *Dry-powder devices* (Turbohaler®, Diskhaler®, Accuhaler®, Clickhaler®) (Fig. 11.7): in these devices the β-agonist or steroid drug is formulated as a dry powder without a propellant. Inspiratory airflow releases the powder from the device so that they are **breath actuated**, and this reduces the problem of coordination of inspiration and inhaler actuation. Some patients find dry-powder devices easier to use but they require an adequate inspiratory flow rate to achieve drug delivery.

• *Nebulisers* (Fig. 11.8): in this form of inhaled therapy, oxygen or compressed air is directed through a narrow hole creating a local negative pressure (Venturi effect) which draws the drug solution into the air stream from a reservoir chamber. The droplets are then impacted against a small sphere, and small particles are carried as an aerosol, whereas larger particles hit the side wall of the

chamber and fall back into the reservoir solution. The aerosol is administered by mask, or via a mouthpiece. Nebulisers are a convenient **means of giving high doses of bronchodilator drugs in acute attacks of asthma** where coordination of inhaler administration may be difficult in a distressed patient. They may also be used for delivering inhaled steroids (e.g. budesonide) in very young children although it is important to realise that properly used dry-powder devices, for example turbohaler, or metered-dose inhalers and spacer devices deliver a greater percentage of the administered dose to the lower airway and are therefore the devices of choice for routine long-term treatment. The danger of patients having machines at home for administration of bronchodilators lies in the fact that they may over-rely on the temporary alleviation of symptoms by nebulised bronchodilators to the detriment of regular anti-inflammatory therapy, and they may delay seeking urgent medical advice during acute severe asthma attacks.

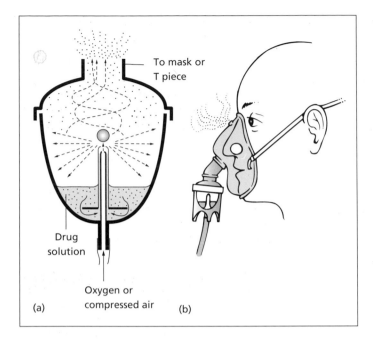

To mask or
T piece

Drug
solution

Oxygen or
compressed air

(a)

(b)

Figure 11.8 Nebuliser treatment. (a) Diagram of typical nebulisation mechanism. (b) Nebuliser mask for administration of high-dose bronchodilator (see text).

ACUTE SEVERE ASTHMA

Some patients with brittle asthma are particularly susceptible to recurrent sudden attacks of severe asthma but any patient with asthma may develop an acute attack under certain circumstances (e.g. viral infection, allergen exposure). It is crucial that all patients with asthma know how to recognise the features of a severe attack and know what action to take. Most of the people who die of acute asthma do so because the severity of the attack was underestimated. Guidelines therefore emphasise the importance of monitoring peak flow measurements during an attack and recognising the features of severe asthma.

Clinical features

- Too breathless to complete sentences in one breath
- Respiratory rate ⩾25 breaths/min
- Heart rate ⩾110 beats/min
- Peak expiratory flow ⩽ 50% of predicted normal or best

Life-threatening features

- Peak expiratory flow <33% of predicted normal or best
- A silent chest, cyanosis or feeble respiratory effort
- Bradycardia or hypotension
- Exhaustion, confusion or coma
- Severe hypoxaemia ($Po_2 < 8\,kPa$ (60 mmHg))
- Normal (5–6 kPa (38–60 mmHg)) or high Pco_2

Immediate management

- *Oxygen*: the highest concentration available should be used. Masks delivering 24 or 28% are not appropriate.
- *High-dose nebulised β-agonist*: for example salbutamol 5 mg or terbutaline 10 mg). This may be repeated after 15–30 minutes if the patient's condition is not improving. Multiple doses from an inhaler should be given with a spacer device if a nebuliser is not available.
- *High-dose systemic steroid*: for example prednisolone 40–50 mg orally, or hydrocortisone 100 mg 6-hourly intravenously, or both, immediately.

If life-threatening features are present add the following.

- *Nebulised ipratropium*: add ipratropium 0.5 mg to the nebulised β-agonist.
- *Intravenous magnesium sulphate*: 1.2–2 g infusion over 20 minutes should be considered for patients with acute severe asthma who have not had a good initial response to nebulised bronchodilator therapy.
- *Intravenous bronchodilators*: some patients with very severe asthma may gain additional benefit from intravenous aminophylline (5 mg/kg loading dose over 20 minutes unless on maintenance oral therapy, then infusion of 0.5 mg/kg/hr). Intravenous β₂-agonists are sometimes used (salbutamol or terbutaline 250 μg over 10 minutes, then infusion of 5 μg/min) but they should be reserved for those patients in whom nebulised therapy cannot be used reliably.

Investigations

Arterial blood gases; urea and electrolyte concentrations; electrocardiogram in older patients; chest X-ray.

Monitoring treatment

Continued vigilance is required. The patient's condition may deteriorate some hours after an initial improvement (e.g. during the night afterwards). Measure and record peak expiratory flow 15–30 minutes after starting treatment and thereafter according to the response (at least 4 times daily measurements). Monitor respiratory rate, pulse, patient's general condition and oxygen saturation frequently. Nursing staff should be asked to call the doctor if there is a deterioration in these signs, and elective transfer of the patient to an intensive therapy unit (ITU) may be advisable so that their condition can be monitored more closely. Intermittent positive pressure ventilation is only rarely necessary but is used when the patient shows signs of exhaustion (e.g. rising P_{CO_2}), failure to maintain oxygenation or deterioration in vital signs.

Management during recovery in hospital and following discharge

The opportunity should be taken to improve the patient's understanding of asthma and its management, and to provide written guidance on future management. Ways of improving the patient's response to worsening asthma should be identified. Most crises resulting in hospital admission are probably preventable. The importance of peak flow measurement in determining treatment changes should be explained. Possible precipitating factors should be identified. Inhaler technique should be checked and performance recorded. If necessary, alternative inhaler devices should be used.

Keypoints

- Asthma is a dynamic heterogenous clinical syndrome, characterised by chronic airway inflammation, airway hyper-responsiveness, symptoms and airways obstruction.
- The clinical diagnosis of asthma should be supported by evidence of variable or reversible airways obstruction on spirometry or peak flow measurements.
- Asthma is multifactorial in origin, arising from a complex interaction of genetic and environmental factors.
- In most patients chronic asthma can be managed satisfactorily by regular inhaled corticosteroids to control airway inflammation and an inhaled bronchodilator to reverse symptoms.
- Instruction in the correct use of an appropriate inhaler device is crucial in the treatment of asthma.
- Treatment of an acute severe attack of asthma involves high flow oxygen, nebulised bronchodilators (e.g salbutamol 5 mg and ipratropium 0.5 mg) and prednisolone 40 mg/day, with vigilance to detect any deterioration.

Further reading

Asthma UK: http://www.asthma.org.uk

British Thoracic Society/Scottish Intercollegiate Guidelines Network. British Guideline on the management of asthma. http://www. brit-thoracic.org-uk

Carlsen KH, Delgado L, DelGiacco S. Diagnosis, prevention and treatment of exercise-related asthma, respiratory and allergic disorders in sports. *Eur Respir Mon* 2005; **10**: 1–105.

Chu EK, Drazen JM. Asthma: one hundred years of treatment and onward. *Am J Respir Crit Care Med* 2005; **171**: 1202–8.

Dolovich MB, Ahrens RC, Hess DR et al. Device selection and outcomes of aerosol therapy: evidence based guidelines of the American College of Chest Physicians/American College of Asthma, Allergy and Immunology. *Chest* 2005; **127**: 335–71.

Global Initiative for Asthma (GINA) http://www.ginasthma.com

Holgate ST, Yang Y, Haitchi HM et al. The genetics of asthma. *Proc Am Thorac Soc* 2006; **3**: 440–3.

Masoli M, Fabian D, Holt S, Beasley R. The global burden of asthma: executive summary of GINA Dissemination Committee report. *Allergy* 2004; **59**: 469–78.

Chapter 12

Chronic obstructive pulmonary disease

Introduction

Chronic obstructive pulmonary disease (COPD) is a major cause of morbidity and mortality worldwide. It has a profound effect on both the quantity and quality of life. In the UK about 1.5 million people have COPD, there are 110 000 admissions to hospital with exacerbations of COPD and 30 000 people die of the disease each year. Mortality has fallen in men but continues to rise in women, reflecting smoking patterns. As the worldwide epidemic of smoking spreads, with increasing smoking rates in China, Africa and Asia it is predicted that COPD will become the third most common cause of death worldwide by 2020. There is an urgent need to improve awareness, prevention and treatment of this disease.

Definitions (Table 12.1)

Chronic obstructive pulmonary disease

COPD is defined as a chronic slowly progressive disorder characterised by **airflow obstruction** that does not change markedly over several months. Although there is some overlap in the features of COPD and asthma, they are separate disorders with different aetiologies, pathologies, natural history and responses to treatment. In asthma, airway

inflammation and hyperreactivity are the key factors giving rise to bronchial muscle contraction and airways obstruction. In COPD, structural changes arising from alveolar destruction by emphysema result in a loss of elastic recoil and a loss of outward traction on the small airways such that they collapse on expiration contributing to the airways obstruction, air trapping and hyperinflation (Figs 12.1 and 12.2).

Chronic bronchitis

Chronic bronchitis is a hypersecretory disorder defined as the presence of **cough productive of sputum on most days for at least 3 months of 2 successive years** in a patient in whom other causes of a chronic cough have been excluded (e.g. tuberculosis, bronchiectasis). The diagnosis is made on the basis of symptoms. The airways of patients with chronic bronchitis show mucous gland hypertrophy and an increased number of goblet cells. The mucous gland hypertrophy may be quantified pathologically by the Reid index which is the ratio of the thickness of the mucous gland layer in the bronchial wall to the total wall thickness. Although chronic bronchitis and obstructive lung disease result from inhaling cigarette smoke, they do not show a clear relationship to each other and are distinct components of the spectrum of COPD.

Table 12.1 Chronic obstructive pulmonary disease (COPD).

Term	Definition	Diagnosis
Chronic bronchitis	Cough and sputum for 3 months of 2 successive years	Symptoms
Airways obstruction	Diffuse airway narrowing with increased resistance to airflow	↓FEV_1/VC
		↓PEF
Asthma	Reversible airways obstruction with airway inflammation and hyper-responsiveness	Bronchodilator and steroid response
Emphysema	Dilatation of the terminal airspaces with destruction of alveoli	Pathology
		CT scan
		↓K_{CO}, ↓T_{LCO}
Respiratory failure	Failure to maintain oxygenation	↓Po_2
		↓O_2 sat
Cor pulmonale	Right heart hypertrophy and failure caused by chronic lung disease	Oedema
		↓JVP
		ECG
		ECHO

CT, computed tomography; ECG, electrocardiogram; ECHO, echocardiography; FEV_1, forced expiratory volume in 1 second; JVP, jugular vein pulse; PEF, peak expiratory flow; VC, vital capacity.

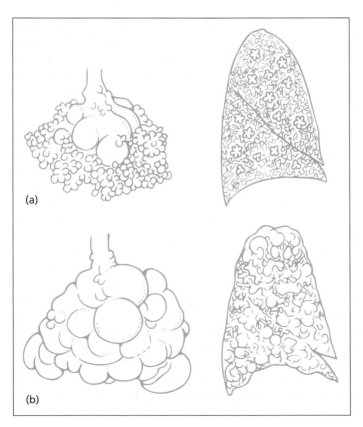

(a)

(b)

Figure 12.1 Emphysema. Diagrammatic view of lobule and whole lung section in (a) centrilobular and (b) panacinar emphysema.

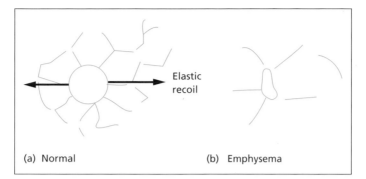

Figure 12.2 Emphysema consists of dilatation of the terminal air spaces of the lungs, distal to the terminal bronchiole with destruction of their walls. Small peripheral airways lack cartilage and depend on the support of the surrounding alveoli to maintain their patency (a). Alveolar destruction in emphysema results in a loss of elastic recoil and a loss of outward traction on the small airways such that they collapse on expiration contributing to the airways obstruction (b).

Mucus hypersecretion is mainly caused by changes in the central airways whereas progressive airways obstruction arises principally from damage to the peripheral airways and alveoli.

Airways obstruction

Airways obstruction is an increased resistance to airflow caused by diffuse airways narrowing. The term denotes a disturbance of physiology as manifest by a **reduced peak expiratory flow, forced expiratory volume in 1 second (FEV_1)** and **FEV_1/ vital capacity (VC) ratio** such that the FEV_1 is less than 80% predicted and the FEV_1/forced vital capacity (FVC) is less than 0.7. The diagnosis is based upon lung function tests. A number of factors contribute to airways obstruction in COPD. Loss of elastic recoil from destruction of alveoli by emphysema is an important factor in producing airway collapse. The airway inflammation in COPD differs from that seen in asthma and is usually the result of tobacco smoke. Accumulation of mucous secretions and superimposed infections may aggravate airways obstruction.

The **degree of reversibility** of the airways obstruction may be assessed by measuring the response to bronchodilator and corticosteroid drugs, and this varies considerably with some patients having a significant reversible component to their disease whereas others have predominantly fixed airways obstruction. The severity of the airways obstruction may be arbitrarily graded according to the FEV_1 value: mild 50–80% of predicted; moderate 30–49% of predicted; severe <30% of predicted.

Emphysema

Emphysema is defined in terms of its pathological features which consist of **dilatation of the terminal air spaces of the lung distal to the terminal bronchiole with destruction of their walls**. Physiologically, emphysema is characterised by a reduction in the transfer factor for carbon monoxide and transfer coefficient. High-resolution computed tomography (CT) scans can demonstrate the parenchymal lung destruction of emphysema. Two main patterns of emphysema are recognised (Fig. 12.1): **centriacinar** (centrilobular) emphysema involves damage around the respiratory bronchioles with preservation of the more distal alveolar ducts and alveoli. Characteristically, it affects the upper lobes and upper parts of the lower lobes of the lung. **Panacinar (panlobular) emphysema** results in distension and destruction of the whole of the acinus, and particularly affects the lower half of the lungs. Although both types of emphysema are related to smoking and may be present together, it is possible that they may arise by different mechanisms and give rise to different patterns of impairment of lung function. Panacinar emphysema is the characteristic feature of patients with α_1-anti-trypsin enzyme deficiency.

Aetiology

Tobacco smoking is the main cause of COPD such that many doctors favour the use of a simple direct term such as **'smoker's lung'** which gives a clear message to the patient about the cause of the disease and the need for smoking cessation. The total dose of tobacco inhaled is important and depends on factors such as **age of starting** smoking, **depth of inhalation** and total **number of cigarettes** smoked (one 'pack year' is defined as the equivalent of 20 cigarettes per day for 1 year).

Although nearly all patients with COPD have smoked heavily, only about 15% of smokers develop COPD, suggesting that additional factors such as genetic susceptibility or other environmental influences play a part. There is a higher prevalence of COPD in **men** than in women, in patients of **lower socioeconomic status** and in **urban** rather than rural areas. The prevalence and mortality rates for COPD are higher in the north and west of England than in the south-east. Many of these geographical and demographic differences simply reflect differences in cigarette smoking habit.

There is strong evidence that COPD may be aggravated by **air pollution** but the role of pollution in the aetiology of COPD appears to be small when compared with that of cigarette smoking. Many **dusty occupations** are associated with the development of chronic bronchitis, and various forms of obstructive airways disease are associated with occupational environments, for example byssinosis in cotton workers, asthma in paint sprayers, obstructive airways disease in farmers (see Chapter 15). However, the contribution of occupation to the development of COPD is small when compared to the dominant effect of cigarette smoking. Nevertheless, exposure to coal dust, cotton dust and grain may be associated with an increased risk for developing COPD.

A variety of **factors in early childhood** have an important influence on the development of obstructive airways disease in adulthood by determining the maximum lung function achieved in adolescence and possibly also the subsequent rate of decline in lung function. Such factors include **passive exposure** to **cigarette smoke** either transplacentally **in utero** or environmentally in the **home. Childhood respiratory illnesses** including respiratory tract infections are also important. Some studies suggest that the presence of **airway responsiveness** predicts an accelerated rate of decline in lung function in smokers. Family and twin studies suggest that **genetic factors** contribute to the differences between individuals in their susceptibility to developing COPD if they smoke, but these factors are poorly defined except in the case of the inherited **deficiency of anti-protease enzymes.** It is thought that emphysema develops as a consequence of destruction of lung tissue by proteolytic digestion resulting from an imbalance between proteases and anti-proteases and between oxidants and anti-oxidants. Genetic deficiency of the principal anti-protease, α_1-anti-trypsin, is associated with the development of severe emphysema at a young age. α_1-anti-trypsin deficiency accounts for fewer than 1% of all cases of COPD but it is possible that other unidentified proteases may be important.

Clinical features and progression

COPD has a wide spectrum of severity. Chronic **cough** and **sputum** production are the clinical manifestations of the mucus hypersecretion of chronic bronchitis which affects about 15% of men and 5% of women in the UK. **Infective exacerbations** of bronchitis are common and are characterised by an increased cough with purulent sputum. Non-typable unencapsulated strains of *Haemophilus influenzae* often colonise the normal upper respiratory tract. In chronic bronchitis disruption of the mucociliary defence mechanism facilitates spread of infection to the bronchial tree, where infection may provoke inflammation and a self-perpetuating vicious circle of inflammation and infection, further compromising pulmonary clearance mechanisms and aggravating airways obstruction. Many exacerbations of chronic bronchitis are associated with infection with respiratory viruses, for example influenza A, but other organisms implicated include *Haemophilus influenzae, Streptococcus pneumoniae, Moraxella catarrhalis* and sometimes 'atypical organisms' such as *Chlamydia pneumoniae*. Extension of

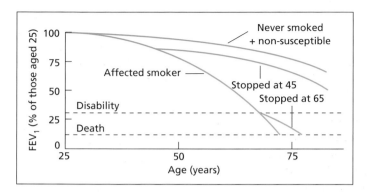

Figure 12.3 Change in FEV_1 with age: effect of smoking and stopping smoking. Non-smokers show a small progressive decline in function with age. By the time disability is noted, ventilatory function is seriously reduced to about one-third of predicted normal values. Many smokers are unaffected by smoking and show the same decline as non-smokers. Some smokers are affected and show a steeper decline. Those affected by smoking can be detected by measurement of FEV_1 many years before they become disabled. Stopping smoking slows the rate of decline. (From Fletcher & Peto, 1977.)

infection into the lung parenchyma gives rise to **bronchopneumonia** (see Chapter 6).

The characteristic feature of airways obstruction and emphysema is gradually progressive **breathlessness** sometimes associated with wheeze. Because of the large pulmonary reserve, patients with a sedentary lifestyle often do not notice breathlessness until a great deal of lung function has been permanently lost. Figure 12.3 illustrates the insidious progressive way in which lung function is lost in COPD and shows the crucial importance of smoking cessation in slowing the rate of decline in FEV_1. Not all patients with chronic bronchitis develop airways obstruction because these are separate, although overlapping, outcomes of smoking-related lung damage. Measurement of FEV_1 and FVC by spirometry is essential in diagnosing airways obstruction, in monitoring the progression of the disease and in assessing the response to treatment. In patients with established airways obstruction, symptoms are often aggravated by exposure to cigarette smoke, cold air, fog, atmospheric pollution and respiratory tract infections. There is generally a **gradual progression of disability** over a period of 10–40 years. This is associated with increasing absence from work, gradual limitation of exercise tolerance and a reduced range of activities. With time, **acute exacerbations** become more alarming and are accompanied by breathlessness at rest and difficulty in expectorating

sputum. Admission to hospital is often required during these episodes.

As lung function deteriorates it is important to monitor oxygen levels by oximetry or arterial blood gas analysis because the symptoms of **respiratory failure** are non-specific, consisting of lethargy, tiredness, loss of energy and general malaise. Hypercapnia may cause headaches particularly on awakening in the mornings. **Cor pulmonale** is a term used to denote right ventricular hypertrophy and right heart failure secondary to chronic lung disease. The clinical features of right heart failure consist of peripheral oedema, elevation of the jugular venous pressure and hepatomegaly sometimes associated with a palpable right ventricular heave and tricuspid regurgitation.

Two main clinical patterns of disturbance may be discerned in patients with advanced COPD, which differ mainly in the extent to which ventilatory drive is preserved in the face of increasing airways obstruction: **'pink puffers'** and **'blue bloaters'** (Fig. 12.4). These represent two extremes of a spectrum and most patients do not fit either pattern completely, but have some features of both. 'Pink puffers' have well-preserved ventilatory drive even in the presence of severe airways obstruction. Dyspnoea is usually intense but blood gases are often maintained in the normal range at rest until the terminal stages of the disease. 'Blue bloaters' have poor ventilatory drive and easily

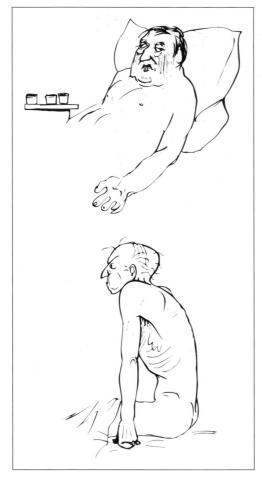

Figure 12.4 'Blue bloater' (above) and 'pink puffer' (below). (Original drawings reproduced by kind permission of Dr R.A.L. Brewis. From *Lecture Notes on Respiratory Disease*, 1st edn.)

drift into respiratory failure with hypercapnia, hypoxaemia and right heart failure, particularly during exacerbations.

It is important to assess the full impact of the disease on all aspects of the patient's life. Breathlessness can be quantified using the **Medical Research Council Dyspnoea Scale**: Grade 1—breathless only on strenuous exertion; Grade 2—breathless when walking up a slight hill; Grade 3—more breathless than contemporaries when walking on level ground; Grade 4—breathless on walking about 100 metres; Grade 5—breathless on dressing or undressing. A number of questionnaires

are available for assessing the overall function and **quality of life**, such as the St George's Hospital Respiratory Questionnaire. **Depression and anxiety** are common and should be sought and treated appropriately. Severe COPD can result in cachexia and loss of muscle mass, and reduced mobility can severely restrict the patient's **social function**. Symptoms, disability and quality of life may be improved by treatments which do not necessarily affect FEV_1.

Investigations

Lung function tests

Spirometry is the most accurate measure of airflow obstruction and is therefore crucial in the diagnosis of COPD. Airflow obstruction is defined as an $FEV_1/VC < 0.7$ and $FEV_1 < 80\%$ predicted. The severity of airflow obstruction can be arbitrarily defined, as mild (FEV_1 50–80% predicted), moderate (FEV_1 30–49% predicted), and severe ($FEV_1 < 30\%$ predicted). Spirometry can also be used to assess the degree of reversibility of the airways obstruction to bronchodilators or corticosteroids but there is considerable variability in the change in FEV_1 in response to the same stimulus from day to day and the overall clinical response to bronchodilators or inhaled corticosteroids cannot be predicted by the response to a reversibility test. **Total lung capacity** and **residual volume** are often elevated signifying hyperinflation and air trapping. **Transfer factor for carbon monoxide** and **transfer coefficient** are typically reduced in emphysema.

Arterial blood gases

Oximetry is useful in measuring oxygen saturation non-invasively but a sample of **arterial blood** is necessary to assess Po_2 and Pco_2 levels.

Radiology (Fig. 12.5)

The **chest X-ray** typically shows hyperinflation of the chest with flattened low hemidiaphragms, an increased retrosternal airspace and a long narrow

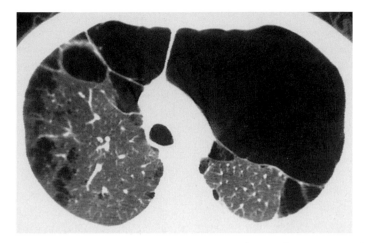

Figure 12.5 This 42-year-old man had smoked 20 cigarettes a day since the age of 14. He presented with a 5-year history of progressive breathlessness and could walk only 100 metres. He had severe airways obstruction with a FEV_1 of 0.5 L, and transfer factor for carbon monoxide and transfer coefficient were reduced to 30% of the predicted values. High-resolution CT shows extensive emphysematous bullae with dilated distal airspaces, cysts and destruction of alveolar architecture. α_1-anti-trypsin levels were unrecordable.

cardiac shadow. The chest X-ray is also an important investigation in excluding additional diagnoses (e.g. lung cancer) and in detecting complications of COPD (e.g. pneumothorax, bronchopneumonia). **High-resolution CT scans** can demonstrate the extent of emphysema and the presence of bullae but are not required for the routine care of patients with COPD.

Sputum microbiology

Antibiotics are often prescribed empirically during exacerbations of COPD based upon a knowledge of the likely organisms. **Sputum culture** may be useful in confirming what organisms are present and in detecting resistance to antibiotics.

General tests

Some patients with chronic hypoxaemia develop polycythaemia with elevated **haemoglobin** levels. **White cell count** may be elevated during infective exacerbations, particularly if infection is not confined to the bronchi but has spread to the lung parenchyma as bronchopneumonia. It is important to assess for any **electrolyte** disturbance in patients with acute exacerbations requiring nebulised

bronchodilator drugs. Patients with cor pulmonale may show features of right ventricular hypertrophy (right axis deviation, dominant R wave in V_1) on **electrocardiography (ECG)** and a dilated hypertrophied ventricle with tricuspid regurgitation on **echocardiography (ECHO)**.

Management

COPD results in a complex pattern of symptoms and disability such that comprehensive management of the disease involves several different components aimed at: (i) **preventing deterioration** in lung function (e.g. smoking cessation); (ii) **alleviating symptoms** (e.g. bronchodilators); (iii) **improving exercise** capacity (e.g. bronchodilators, rehabilitation); (iv) **improving quality of life** (e.g. rehabilitation); (v) **reducing frequency of exacerbations** (e.g. influenza vaccination, inhaled corticosteroids); and (vi) **treating secondary complications** such as malnutrition, cor pulmonale, muscle wasting and depression. Although FEV_1 is a crucial measurement in diagnosing COPD and in defining its severity it is a less useful outcome index when assessing the success of treatment. Important improvements in breathlessness, exercise capacity and quality of life can be achieved by treatments which do not significantly increase FEV_1. In COPD breathlessness on exercise relates more to the physiological process of **dynamic hyperinflation** than to FEV_1. In the normal person at the end of expiration when the lungs are at functional residual capacity, the tendency for the lungs to contract down (elastic recoil) and for the chest wall to spring out are in balance and no effort is required to maintain this lung volume. In COPD there is airways obstruction and reduced expiratory flow such that the lungs become hyperinflated with an increased residual volume and functional residual capacity with the result that the lungs are in a stretched state, and breathing from this higher lung volume requires more effort. This hyperinflation is worsened during exercise resulting in breathlessness. Treatment may reduce dynamic hyperventilation on exercise without significantly changing FEV_1.

Smoking cessation (see Chapter 20) is the most important treatment in preventing loss of lung function in COPD. The pharmacological treatment of COPD depends on the severity of the disease and the level of symptoms, and needs to be integrated into a comprehensive overall management plan (Fig. 12.6).

Drug treatment (see also Chapter 11)

Bronchodilators

β_2-agonists

Short-acting β_2-agonists, such as salbutamol and terbutaline, relax bronchial smooth muscle by stimulation of β-adrenoreceptors. **Long-acting β_2-agonists**, such as salmeterol and formoterol, give more prolonged relief of symptoms with a duration of action of about 12 hours. **Short-acting anticholinergic drugs**, such as ipratropium, produce bronchodilatation by blocking the bronchosconstrictor effect of vagal nerve stimulation of bronchial smooth muscle. Tiotropium is a **long-acting anticholinergic drug** which has greater affinity and a slower rate of dissociation from muscarinic receptors than ipratropium, with a once daily dosage regimen and an important effect in improvement of key clinical outcomes in COPD. β_2-agonists and anti-cholinergic drugs act in different ways such that combinations of both drugs give additional benefits. **Methylxanthines** such as aminophylline and theophyllines have a number of effects including cyclic adenosine monophosphate (cAMP) stimulation of β-adrenoceptors by inhibiting the metabolism of cAMP by the enzyme phosphodiesterase.

Corticosteroids

The airways inflammation of COPD differs from that in asthma in that it is predominantly a neutrophilic inflammation caused by tobacco smoke and is less responsive to corticosteroid therapy. The role for **inhaled corticosteroids** (e.g. beclometasone, budesonide, fluticasone) in COPD is, therefore, very different from that in asthma. Inhaled steroids seem to be ineffective in mild COPD but in moderate and severe COPD they reduce the rate of exacerbations. **Oral corticosteroids** have an important role in the treatment of exacerbations of COPD. Sometimes a trial of prednisolone 30 mg/day for 14 days is given to assess the degree of reversibility of airways obstruction. This is particularly intended to differentiate patients who have asthma from patients with COPD. However in COPD an oral corticosteroid reversibility test does not predict response to inhaled corticosteroid therapy.

Mucolytics

Mucolytics are drugs which increase the expectoration of sputum by reducing its viscosity. Carbocisteine can reduce the frequency of exacerbations in some patients with COPD who have a chronic productive cough.

Drug treatments are often prescribed in a stepwise fashion in accordance with the level of the patient's symptoms and the severity of the airways obstruction. Several different factors (e.g. symptoms, exacerbation rate, exercise capacity, quality of life) need to be considered in judging the effect of treatment and drugs should be stopped if they are not proving beneficial or if they are causing adverse effects (Fig. 12.6). Patients with mild COPD are often managed by smoking cessation and use of

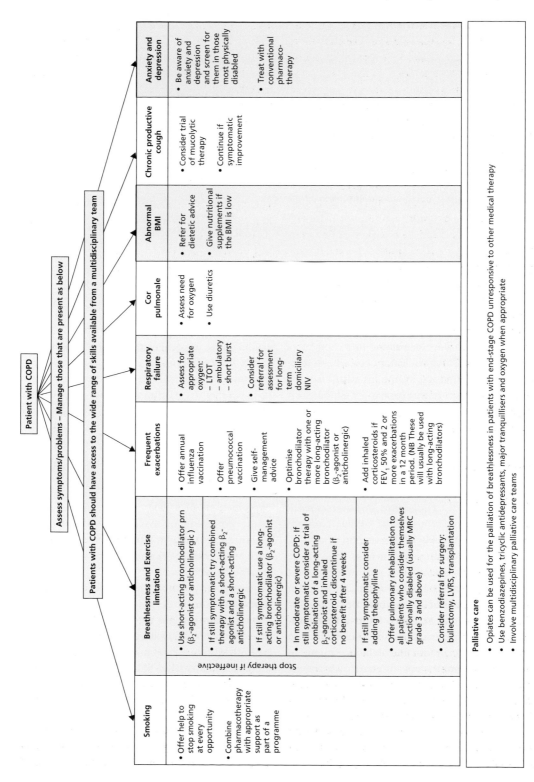

Figure 12.6 The management of patients with stable COPD (Reproduced with permission from the British Thoracic Society guidelines on the Management of COPD (*Thorax* 2004; **59**: Suppl. 1).

Table 12.2 Treatment of severe exacerbations of COPD.

Tests

Chest X-ray, oximetry, arterial blood gases, peak flow, ECG, sputum culture, blood count, urea, electrolytes

Treatment

- Bronchodilators, for example nebulised **salbutamol** 2.5–5 mg and **ipratropium** 250–500 mcg; repeat as needed and continue 4–6 hourly
- Steroids: **prednisolone** 30 mg/day orally for 5–14 days
- Antibiotics, for example **amoxicillin** 500 mg t.i.d. orally or intravenously. Check previous sputum microbiology and consider ciprofloxacin, clarithromycin, co-amoxiclav if needed
- Oxygen: aim for O_2 sat. > 90% without provoking hypercapnia and acidaemia using **controlled oxygen therapy** (e.g. 24% Venturi mask) as necessary
- Ventilatory support: **non-invasive ventilation** if hypercapnic with pH < 7.35 or endotracheal ventilation in ITU if appropriate
- Additional treatments: consider need for diuretics, for example **furosemide** 40 mg intravenously if in cardiac failure; or venesection if severe polycythaemia (e.g. packed cell volume >58%)
- Assisted early discharge services

a short-acting bronchodilator 'as required'. In contrast many patients with advanced COPD will derive benefit from an intensive regimen combining inhaled steroids, long-acting bronchodilators and short-acting bronchodilators, but will still have ongoing disability and symptoms which can be helped by non-pharmacological interventions such as pulmonary rehabilitation.

Antibiotics

In some cases, exacerbations of COPD are associated with infections with viruses or with bacteria such as *Haemophilus influenzae*, *Streptococcus pneumoniae* or *Moraxella catarrhalis*. Although **amoxicillin** has a reasonably good spectrum of activity against many of these organisms, 15–20% of *Haemophilus influenzae* and many strains of *Moraxella catarrhalis* are resistant to **amoxicillin** so that other antibiotics such as **co-amoxiclav** (amoxicillin and clavulanic acid), **trimethoprim**, **ciprofloxacin**, **tetracycline** or **clarithromycin** may be needed. Sputum microbiology is useful in guiding antibiotic therapy. In many cases exacerbations of COPD seem to arise as a result of spontaneous deterioration in the disease process or are provoked by non-infectious events such as air pollution, smoking or adverse weather conditions. It may be difficult to judge the importance of using an antibiotic as one element alongside use of

bronchodilators, steroids, oxygen and sputum clearance techniques in exacerbations of COPD (Table 12.2). There is evidence of the beneficial effect of antibiotics in hastening the rate of recovery **in severe exacerbations** of COPD associated with increasing cough, sputum production and dyspnoea but there is no definite evidence of the benefit of antibiotics in mild exacerbations. Pneumococcal vaccination and annual **influenza vaccination** are recommended for patients with COPD.

Exacerbations of COPD

Exacerbations of COPD are characterised by an acute worsening of symptoms with increased breathlessness, sputum production and sputum purulence. They may occur spontaneously or as a result of infections or air pollution. Patients can be taught to recognise the onset of an exacerbation and to institute a **self-management plan** whereby they increase the dose and frequency of bronchodilator medication and start a course of oral prednisolone and an antibiotic, according to a predetermined plan. Mild exacerbations can be **managed at home** but patients with severe exacerbations require **admission to hospital**. Deciding whether a patient can be managed at home requires an overall assessment of the severity of the COPD (e.g. baseline FEV_1, oxygen saturation, exercise capacity), the home circumstances (e.g.

family support, able to cope), and key adverse features which indicate a severe exacerbation (e.g. confusion, cyanosis, severe respiratory distress). Patients admitted to hospital should have a chest X-ray, oximetry, arterial blood gas measurement, an electrocardiograph and full blood count and urea and electrolyte measurements. Culture of sputum may be useful in guiding antibiotic therapy. Bronchodilator therapy is usually given by nebuliser using a combination of **salbutamol** 2.5—5 mg and **ipratropium** 250–500 mcg with **prednisolone** 30–40 mg/day for 5–14 days. **Antibiotics** are indicated if there is sputum purulence or if the patient has severe COPD. The aim of oxygen therapy is to achieve an oxygen saturation >90% without provoking critical hypercapnia and respiratory acidosis. **Non-invasive ventilation (NIV)** is now the standard treatment for patients with hypercapnia and acidosis (pH < 7.35) as it significantly improves mortality in these patients (see below). The intensity and duration of treatment is adapted in accordance with the severity of the exacerbation and the rate of improvement, and many patients will be suitable for **early assisted discharge home** with 'hospital at home' support.

Pulmonary rehabilitation

Pulmonary rehabilitation is a multidisciplinary programme of care for patients with COPD that is individually tailored and designed to optimise the patient's physical and social performance and autonomy. Typically a pulmonary rehabilitation programme involves the skills of doctors, respiratory nurse specialists, physiotherapists, dieticians, social workers and occupational therapists. Many patients with COPD are in a vicious cycle of breathlessness, reduced physical activity and deconditioning of skeletal muscles, with resultant loss of social contact and autonomy. Pulmonary rehabilitation can break this vicious cycle and improve quality of life. The key components of a rehabilitation programme need to be adjusted to meet the needs of the individual patient, but typically include:

• *Smoking cessation*: advice, encouragement and support in achieving and maintaining smoking cessation (see Chapter 20).

• *Optimising drug treatment*: ensuring that the patient is taking a comprehensive treatment regimen, with a good inhaler technique.

• *Education* of the patient and family about the nature and cause of the disease and its management. The programme should include aspects such as how and when to take medications, the benefits of exercise, the importance of smoking cessation, and the use of techniques such as breathing control, relaxation and anxiety management. Patients who are vulnerable to exacerbations can be taught to recognise the onset of symptoms of an exacerbation and instructed to start a course of prednisolone and to increase their use of bronchodilator drugs, with an antibiotic for purulent sputum.

• *Exercise training*: breathless patients often reduce their level of exercise and lose general fitness and muscle mass which cause a vicious cycle of deteriorating exercise capacity. Exercise training (e.g. walking, cycling) can counteract muscle atrophy and improve fitness. Improvement in lower limb function may help walking, and arm training improves performance of day-to-day tasks such as lifting, dressing, washing and brushing hair, for example. Typically an exercise training programme involves three supervised aerobic exercise sessions per week over a period of 2 months. Such a programme improves functional walking distance, symptoms and quality of life.

• *Breathing control techniques* involve pursed lip breathing, slower deeper respirations and better coordination of breathing patterns. Physiotherapy techniques such as postural drainage, chest percussion and forced expiratory techniques may be useful in patients who have difficulty expectorating secretions.

• *Psychosocial support*: patients with advanced disability may have difficulty in performing daily tasks such as climbing stairs, shopping and washing, and may benefit from assessment by an occupational therapist with regard to home aids such as stairlifts and bath aids. Depression and social isolation are common and can be helped by psychological support focusing on restoring coping skills. Patient self-help groups may be useful. Assessment by a social worker allows the patient to obtain appropriate allowances, such as disability or mobility allowances, from government agencies.

• *Nutrition*: Poor nutrition is common in patients with advanced COPD and is associated with poor overall health status and an increased mortality. Patients with COPD are often underweight because of the increased work of breathing, the systemic effects of inflammatory cytokines and decreased food intake from anorexia and breathlessness. Some patients, in contrast, are overweight because of reduced activity and overeating. The patient's weight and body mass index should be measured and appropriate dietary advice given.

Surgery

A small number of patients with COPD may benefit from surgery. **Lung transplantation** is an option, particularly for patients with emphysema caused by α_1-anti-trypsin deficiency, although lack of donor organs severely limits the application of this procedure. **Bullectomy** may be appropriate where a large bulla is compressing surrounding viable lung. In recent years **volume reduction surgery** is an option for selected patients with severe disability. In emphysema, destruction of the alveoli results in a loss of elastic recoil with collapse of small airways on expiration and hyperinflation of the lungs with flattening of the diaphragm. Volume reduction surgery aims to resect functionally useless areas of lung thereby reducing the overall volume of the lungs in order to restore elastic recoil so that there is an increased outward traction on the small airways, relief of compression of normal lung and restoration of more normal diaphragmatic and thoracic contours allowing better respiratory motion during breathing. Patients whose emphysema preferentially affects the upper lobes may be the most suitable patients for this procedure. In certain patients lung function, exercise performance and quality of life are improved but the benefit tends to decline with time.

Oxygen therapy

Oxygen delivery to the tissues of the body depends upon the inspired oxygen concentration, ventilation, gas exchange and distribution in the circulation. **Oxygen therapy** should be prescribed with due attention to the **dose** and **method of administration** and with careful **monitoring of its effects**. It is also important to optimise oxygen transport to the tissues by ensuring adequate haemoglobin level, cardiac output and tissue perfusion. It is important to understand that shortness of breath does not necessarily imply shortage of oxygen. Oximetry and arterial blood gas analysis are essential in initiating, monitoring and adjusting oxygen therapy.

Method of administration

Air, at sea level, contains about 21% oxygen. An inspired concentration of 100% oxygen can only be achieved in the context of **artificial ventilation** in an intensive therapy unit (ITU) or with apparatus which provides a complete seal from the outside air and a non-return valve. High concentrations (e.g. 60–90%) can be administered via a tight-fitting face mask attached to a **reservoir bag**, although there is a potential for rebreathing of exhaled carbon dioxide. Concentrations of about 40–60% can be achieved with **simple masks in which oxygen is supplied directly to the mask space** (Fig. 12.7). The effective concentration achieved depends upon the oxygen flow and on the pattern of breathing because some air from the room is drawn into the mask diluting the oxygen concentration. **Nasal cannulae** (prongs) are the most convenient way of administering oxygen because, in contrast to masks, they are relatively unobtrusive and do not interfere with speech or eating. They are usually well tolerated and kept in place continuously so that oxygen therapy is not interrupted during sleeping or eating. The oxygen concentration administered via nasal cannulae varies not only with the oxygen flow rate but also with the patient's ventilatory rate, tidal volume and degree of mouth breathing, so that it cannot be accurately predicted and provides a relatively 'uncontrolled' form of oxygen therapy. If an accurate and constantly controlled concentration of oxygen is required then a **fixed performance Venturi mask** is necessary. Oxygen flow from

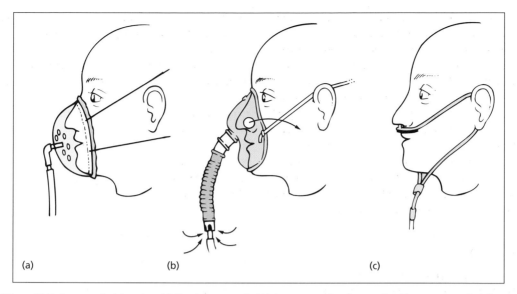

Figure 12.7 Oxygen administration. (a) Simple uncontrolled high-concentration face mask with oxygen supplied directly to the mask space. (b) Fixed performance Venturi mask delivering a controlled dose of low-concentration oxygen. (c) Nasal cannulae delivering an uncontrolled level of oxygen in a convenient continuous manner.

a specifically designed pinhole orifice creates a local negative pressure which entrains a constant proportion of room air through side ports at the base of the mask (small arrows, Fig. 12.7b). A selection of masks giving 24, 28 and 35% oxygen is available and the concentration delivered is dependent upon the size of the pinhole and the designs of the apertures and is relatively independent of the patient's pattern of breathing. Humidification of inspired oxygen is only needed when it is delivered directly to the trachea or at high flow rates, otherwise the oropharynx provides adequate humidification.

Acute oxygen therapy

High-concentration oxygen should be given empirically in cases of cardiac or respiratory arrest or in acute life-threatening situations (e.g. acute severe asthma). Patients with established respiratory failure who have chronically raised P_{CO_2} (type 2 respiratory failure) become unresponsive to the carbon dioxide stimulus to ventilation and rely increasingly on hypoxaemia to maintain the drive to breathe. If they are given high concentrations of oxygen they breathe less and underbreathing

results in increasing hypercapnia, acidosis, narcosis and ultimately respiratory depression. Uncontrolled oxygen therapy poses a risk to a subset of patients with COPD (notably 'blue bloaters' with hypercapnic (type 2) respiratory failure), although this risk has often been exaggerated and must be balanced against the threat of hypoxaemia.

Because of the shape of the oxyhaemoglobin dissociation curve, there is little benefit in increasing the patient's oxygen saturation above about 90% or the P_{O_2} above about 8 kPa (60 mmHg). In treating patients with acute exacerbations of COPD, therefore, the aim of oxygen therapy is to correct hypoxaemia to a $P_{O_2} > 8$ kPa (60 mmHg) or oxygen saturation >90% without provoking critical hypercapnia and respiratory acidosis. Very often this can be achieved by measuring oximetry with the patient breathing air and then giving controlled oxygen therapy, for example using a 24 or 28% fixed performance Venturi mask to achieve an oxygen saturation above 90%. Arterial blood gases are then analysed when the patient has been breathing the required amount of oxygen for about 30 minutes. If the P_{CO_2} is below 6 kPa (45 mmHg) then it is safe to transfer to nasal cannulae using oximetry to determine the flow rate required (e.g. 1–2 L/min) to maintain oxygen saturation just above 90%. Judicious use of oximetry and measurement of arterial blood gases under precisely judged circumstances (e.g. when the patient has reached steady state on the required concentration of oxygen as judged by oximetry) can limit the need for repeated arterial blood sampling. It is essential to document carefully the amount of oxygen being breathed when measuring arterial gases. Avoid measuring gases immediately after the patient has received nebulised drugs using high-flow oxygen. Sometimes there is concern about using high-flow oxygen (e.g. 6–8 L/min) to nebulise bronchodilator drugs in patients with hypercapnia and occasionally air is used to nebulise these drugs. However, nebulising drugs using air during acute exacerbations of COPD may leave the patient dangerously hypoxic and it is probably better to continue using oxygen 6–8 L/min to nebulise the drug but to limit the nebulisation time strictly to 10–15 minutes so that the patient is not exposed to the risk of either hypoxia or prolonged high-concentration oxygen.

Ventilatory support

Many patients admitted to hospital with an exacerbation of COPD and acute hypercapnic respiratory failure will improve rapidly with initial medical treatments and controlled oxygen therapy. In those with persistant hypercapnia and acidosis (pH < 7.35) despite medical therapy NIV is the treatment of choice as it reduces mortality and the need for intubation. It is delivered via a tight-fitting mask strapped in place over the nose and mouth, connected to a specifically designed ventilating machine. The spontaneous respiratory efforts of the patient may be used to trigger the ventilator to deliver additional tidal volume under positive pressure. Alternatively, mandatory controlled ventilation may be delivered to the patient with a set tidal volume, inflation pressure and ventilatory rate and no patient effort is required. If the patient fails to improve on NIV, or is not suitable for NIV, then a respiratory stimulant such as intravenous **doxapram** may be useful but

invasive ventilation (i.e. endotracheal intubation and ventilation on ITU) should be considered.

In some cases the patient's underlying disease has progressed to a stage where mechanical ventilation in ITU is unlikely to be successful and a palliative approach towards relief of symptoms is more appropriate than futile treatment which may merely prolong the process of dying to the distress of the patient and his or her relatives.

Long-term oxygen therapy

Patients with COPD and chronic hypoxaemia have a poor prognosis with a mortality rate of about 50% within 3 years. The clinical features of hypoxaemia are non-specific, and periodic measurement of oxygen saturation by oximetry is useful in detecting these patients. Hypoxaemia is a powerful stimulus to pulmonary artery vasoconstriction which if persistent provokes pulmonary hypertension, right ventricular hypertrophy and right heart failure (cor pulmonale). In the early 1980s two major studies, the American Nocturnal Oxygen Therapy Trial (NOTT) and the British Medical Research Council (MRC) Study, showed that the administration of oxygen for at least 15 hours/day (preferably longer) improved survival in patients with severe airflow obstruction (FEV_1 < 1.5 L) and hypoxaemia (Po_2 < 7.3 kPa (55 mmHg)) who had peripheral oedema.

Prescribing criteria
Long-term home oxygen therapy is indicated for **non-smoking patients with severe COPD (FEV_1 < 1.5 L) and persistent hypoxaemia (Po_2 < 7.3 kPa (55 mmHg))**. Many patients who are hypoxaemic during an exacerbation will recover over a few weeks and will not require long-term oxygen. Arterial blood gases should therefore be measured on two occasions, at least 3 weeks apart, during a stable phase before diagnosing persistent hypoxaemia. Patients with more borderline oxygen levels (7.3–8.0 kPa (55–60 mmHg)) who have elevated haematocrit or features of cor pulmonale such as oedema are also likely to benefit from long-term oxygen. The oxygen is usually given via nasal cannulae at a flow rate of about

2 L/min but the dose required and mode of administration should be decided by a specialist in the context of the patient's arterial blood gas measurement.

Oxygen concentrator

Long-term home oxygen therapy is often provided from an oxygen concentrator. This is an electrically powered machine that separates oxygen from the ambient air using a molecular sieve. The machine is installed in the patient's house and plastic tubing relays oxygen to points such as the bedroom and living room. Providing oxygen cylinders to the patient's home for long-term oxygen therapy is impractical and much more expensive than installation of an oxygen concentrator. The patient and family should be warned not to smoke in the presence of oxygen because of the risk of causing a fire. It is essential that the patient understands that the main aim of long-term oxygen therapy is to improve prognosis (reduce mortality rate) rather than to alleviate symptoms and that it is necessary to comply with oxygen therapy for at least 15 hours/day. The patient achieves this by using oxygen during sleep at night and while ordinary domestic activities are performed during the day.

Ambulatory oxygen

Ambulatory oxygen may be appropriate for patients who are active enough to leave the home regularly, who demonstrate a fall in oxygen saturation of more than 4% to below 90% on exercise and who show symptomatic benefit from oxygen in terms of walking distance or reduced breathlessness. It is given using a refillable portable container of liquid oxygen. **Short burst oxygen** is the use of oxygen for short periods to relieve dyspnoea after exercise. In these circumstances the patients typically breathes oxygen from a cylinder for a few minutes after exercise around the house. However the benefit of this form of oxygen therapy is not clearly established.

In the UK home oxygen is now supplied by designated companies who install and maintain all forms of oxygen systems in the patient's home after the patient has undergone specialist assessment. This assessment involves the measurement of arterial blood gases over time to confirm persistent hypoxaemia, and repeat measurements whilst breathing oxygen to determine the required dose and delivery system. Oximetry is used to measure desaturation on exercise, and the patient's exercise performance can be assessed using tests such as the 6-minute walk test (records the distance the patient can walk in 6 minutes) to determine if ambulatory oxygen may be indicated. There is an important role for respiratory nurse specialists in undertaking oxygen assessments and in educating and supporting patients on home oxygen.

Hypoxia during air travel

Patients with lung disease are vulnerable to developing hypoxia when travelling by plane. Commercial aircraft routinely fly at about 38 000 feet (11 400 m) and are pressurised to a cabin altitude of 8000 feet (2438 m) The reduced partial pressure of oxygen at this altitude is equivalent to breathing 15% oxygen at sea level, and causes the Po_2 of a healthy passenger to fall to between 7.0 and 8.5 kPa (52–64 mmHg). Although this doesn't usually cause symptoms or problems for most passengers it can produce critical hypoxia for patients with lung disease. Pre-flight assessment should include an overall assessment of the patient's condition and treatment with particular regard to dyspnoea, exercise capacity, previous flying experience, spirometry and oxygenation. If the oxygen saturation is >95% then in-flight oxygen is not required. If oxygen. saturation is <92% supplementary in-flight oxygen is usually prescribed at a rate of 2–4 L/min by nasal cannulae. If the oxygen saturation is between 92 and 95% then further assessment is recommended. This may include a **hypoxic challenge test** during which arterial blood gases are measured when the patient has been breathing 15% oxygen for 20 minutes, and in-flight oxygen is usually recommended if the Po_2 falls below 7.4 kPa (55 mmHg).

'Hospital at home' for COPD

Novel ways of managing patients with acute exacerbations of COPD are being developed. In some cases admission to hospital can be avoided by undertaking an initial assessment, including a chest X-ray, arterial blood gas analysis and spirometry, in an **acute respiratory assessment service** and selecting patients who can be safely managed at home with provision of oxygen, nebulised bronchodilators, antibiotics and steroids, with daily domiciliary visits by trained nurse specialists who monitor progress and provide education and reassurance. For other patients **assisted early discharge** is more appropriate whereby after initial treatment and stabilisation in hospital ongoing care is provided to the patient in their own home. Such **'hospital at home'** services are safe, effective and very popular with patients.

Keypoints

- Smoking-related COPD is a major cause of morbidity and mortality worldwide.
- Spirometry is essential in assessing airways obstruction (FEV_1/FVC ratio $\leqslant 0.7$) in COPD.
- Smoking cessation is the most important intervention in reducing the rate of progression of COPD.
- Combinations of inhaled β_2-agonist end anticholinergic bronchodilators and corticosteroids improve symptoms, exercise capacity and quality of life.
- During exacerbations of COPD patients who remain hypercapnic and acidotic (pH < 7.35) despite nebulised bronchodilators, systemic steroids, antibiotics and controlled oxygen therapy should be treated with NIV.
- Pulmonary rehabilitation improves the patient's physical and social performance and quality of life.
- Long-term oxygen therapy at home improves the prognosis of patients with COPD who have persistent hypoxia ($Po_2 < 7.3$ kPa (55 mmHg)).

Further reading

British Thoracic Society standards of care committee. Non-invasive ventilation in acute respiratory failure. *Thorax* 2002; **57**: 192–211.

British Thoracic Society standards of care committee. Managing passengers with respiratory disease planning air travel. *Thorax* 2002; **57**: 289–304.

Celli BR, MacNee W. Standards for the diagnosis and treatment of patients with COPD: a summary of the ATS/ERS position paper. *Eur Respir J* 2004; **23**: 932–46.

Chronic obstructive pulmonary disease: national clinical guideline on management of COPD in adults in primary and secondary care. *Thorax* 2004; **59** (Suppl. 1): 1–232. www.nice.org.uk/CG012NICEguideline

Fletcher C, Peto R. The natural history of chronic airflow obstruction. *BMJ* 1977; **1**: 1645.

Gibson GJ. Oxygen treatment at home. *BMJ* 2006; **332**: 191–2

Global initiative for chronic obstructive lung disease. Global strategy for the diagnosis, management, and prevention of chronic obstructive pulmonary disease. www.goldcopd.com

Ram FSF, Wedzicha JA, Wright J, Greenstone M. Hospital at home for patients with acute exacerbations of chronic obstructive pulmonary disease: systematic review of evidence. *BMJ* 2004; **329**: 315.

Chapter 13

Carcinoma of the lung

Introduction

Lung cancer is the most common cause of cancer death in the world with more than one million deaths occurring yearly. In the UK it kills about 34 000 people each year and it has overtaken breast cancer as the leading cause of cancer death in women. It is a lethal disease with only 20% of patients surviving 1 year, and only 5% surviving 5 years from diagnosis. The vast majority of lung cancers are caused by smoking, and smoking prevention and smoking cessation are the crucial issues in dealing with this major public health problem.

Aetiology (Table 13.1)

The epidemic spread of lung cancer in the 20th century followed about 20 years after increases in **tobacco-smoking** habits (Fig. 13.1). The commercial manufacture of cigarettes started around 1900 and smoking soon became popular amongst men. At that time lung cancer was a very rare disease. By the end of the 1940s about 70% of men and 40% of women smoked. Doctors then started to be aware of an increasing incidence of lung cancer and noticed that the patients were smokers. By 1950 an epidemic of lung cancer had become apparent and studies, such as those of Doll and Hill in the 1950s, established the causative link between smoking and lung cancer. Doll and Hill

Table 13.1 Aetiology of carcinoma of the lung.

- Tobacco smoking
- Passive smoking
- Genetic factors
- Urban environment
- Ionising radiation (e.g. radon gas)
- Asbestos exposure
- Diffuse lung fibrosis (e.g. fibrosing alveolitis)
- Lack of dietary fruit and vegetables

studied the smoking habits and cause of death of UK doctors and showed a significant and steadily rising incidence of deaths from lung cancer as the amount of tobacco smoked increased. At that time 83% of doctors had smoked but thereafter the medical profession were the first to put research into practice, by stopping smoking! In the early 1960s the Royal College of Physicians of London and the Surgeon General of the USA published their landmark reports documenting the causal relationship between smoking and lung cancer. The risk of death from bronchial carcinoma increases by a factor roughly equal to the number of cigarettes smoked per day. For example, a man smoking 30 cigarettes/day has over 30 times the risk of dying from lung cancer than a man who has never smoked. On stopping smoking, excess risk is approximately halved every 5 years thereafter. Smoking has decreased in popularity such that now about 29% of men and 28% of women smoke. Reflecting these changes, lung cancer mortality rates have

Chapter 14

Interstitial lung disease

Introduction

Clinical presentation

The terms 'interstitial lung disease' and 'diffuse parenchymal lung disease' are imprecise clinical terms used to refer to a diverse range of diseases which affect the alveoli and septal interstitium of the lung, and which may progress to diffuse lung fibrosis. Patients with these diseases typically present with progressive **breathlessness**, a dry cough, lung **crackles** and diffuse **infiltrates on chest X-ray**. Lung function tests usually show a restrictive defect (reduced total lung capacity and vital capacity (VC), with normal forced expiratory volume in 1 second/VC (FEV_1/VC) ratio, **impaired gas diffusion** (reduced transfer factor) and **hypoxaemia** with hypocapnia.

Differential diagnosis

At presentation the differential diagnosis includes a number of other diseases such as infective pneumonia, pulmonary oedema, bronchiectasis and malignancy (e.g. alveolar cell carcinoma). The overall context of the disease is important and exclusion of other diseases may require further investigations (e.g. echocardiography) or observing the response to treatments (e.g. antibiotics, diuretics). Once the clinical features suggest interstitial lung disease a careful search for potential causes is undertaken.

Particular attention is paid to any environmental **antigens** (e.g. budgerigar), **toxins** (e.g. paraquat) or **dusts** (e.g. asbestos) that the patient encounters in his or her **occupational** or **home environment**. **Systemic diseases** (e.g. rheumatoid disease) commonly involve the lung parenchyma and many **drugs** can cause lung fibrosis (e.g. amiodarone, nitrofurantoin, bleomycin) or eosinophilic reactions in the alveoli (e.g. sulphonamides, naproxen).

Investigations

After a detailed clinical assessment, chest X-ray and lung function tests the next key investigation is high-resolution computed tomography (CT) which gives precise information about the extent and pattern of the disease. In some cases this allows a diagnosis to be made with reasonable certainty but it may be useful to proceed to biopsy of the lung parenchyma to study the histological pattern of the disease. Small samples can be obtained by **transbronchial biopsy** of the lung parenchyma through a flexible bronchoscope (Fig. 14.1). Larger samples can be obtained by **surgical biopsy** under general anaesthesia either by **thoracotomy** or by **video-assisted thoracoscopy**. In many cases the histological features are characteristic of a particular disease (e.g. granulomas in sarcoidosis or extrinsic allergic alveolitis; tumour cells in lymphangitis carcinomatosa), but in advanced disease the histology may show non-specific lung fibrosis without

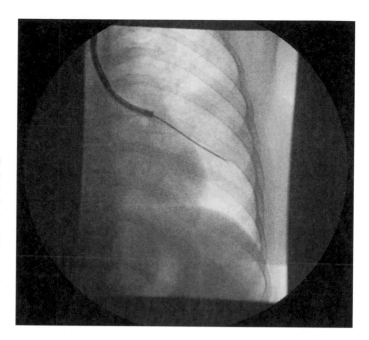

Figure 14.1 Transbronchial lung biopsy. A small specimen of lung parenchyma can be obtained by passing a biopsy forceps through a flexible bronchoscope, usually under radiological guidance, into the lung periphery. A sample of lung tissue is obtained by biopsying between two limbs in a branching small bronchus. There is a small risk of causing haemorrhage or pneumothorax, so the patient's condition and lung function should be adequate to tolerate these complications.

clues to its aetiology. **Bronchoalveolar lavage** may be performed through the bronchoscope at the same time as transbronchial biopsy. Aliquots of saline are instilled via the bronchoscope which is held in a wedged position in a subsegmental bronchus, and fluid is then aspirated for cell analysis. A lymphocytic alveolitis is characteristic of sarcoidosis, for example. Many of these diseases are characterised in their early stages by an inflammatory alveolitis, which is responsive to corticosteroids, whereas in the later stages there may be irreversible lung fibrosis.

Careful clinical investigation of patients presenting with features of interstitial lung disease aims to move from this imprecise clinical label to a diagnosis of a specific disease process (Fig. 14.2).

Idiopathic pulmonary fibrosis

Idiopathic pulmonary fibrosis (IPF) (cryptogenic fibrosing alveolitis) is the classic example of a diffuse fibrotic lung disease. It is a serious disease which kills about 1000 people each year in the UK. It is more common in men (**male/female ratio 2:1**) and in the older age groups (**mean age 67 years**). It presents with the typical features of an interstitial

lung disease as progressive dyspnoea, dry cough, crackles, restrictive defect in lung function and reticulonodular **infiltrates on chest X-ray** (Fig. 14.3). About 60–70% have clubbing. The aetiology is unknown but it appears to be the result of a failure of repair of lung tissue, whereby injury culminates in fibrosis rather than a controlled inflammatory and healing process. A possible association with previous exposure to environmental dusts (e.g. metal or wood dust) has been found in some epidemiological studies, cigarette smoking may be a co-factor for the initiation of the disease, and about 30% of patients have autoantibodies (e.g. rheumatoid factor, anti-nuclear factor) in their serum. Lung biopsy shows a characteristic pattern of '**usual interstitial pneumonia**' with a heterogenous appearance such that there are alternating areas of normal lung, interstitial inflammation, fibrosis and honeycombing. The changes are more severe subpleurally. **High-resolution CT** scan typically shows evidence of advanced fibrosis with extensive areas of **reticulation and honeycombing** in a predominantly lower zone, subpleural distribution with minimal evidence of inflammation as **ground glass opacities** (Fig. 14.4). Patients are usually treated with a combination

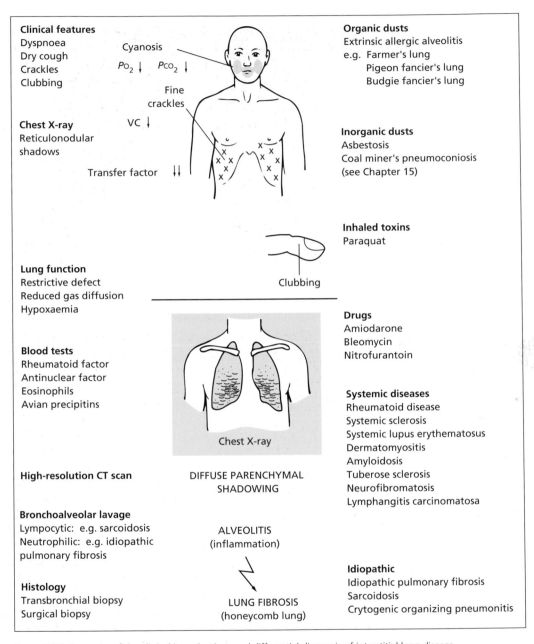

Clinical features
Dyspnoea
Dry cough
Crackles
Clubbing

Cyanosis

$Po_2 \downarrow$ $Pco_2 \downarrow$

Fine crackles

Chest X-ray
Reticulonodular shadows

$VC \downarrow$

Transfer factor $\downarrow\downarrow$

Lung function
Restrictive defect
Reduced gas diffusion
Hypoxaemia

Blood tests
Rheumatoid factor
Antinuclear factor
Eosinophils
Avian precipitins

High-resolution CT scan

Bronchoalveolar lavage
Lympocytic: e.g. sarcoidosis
Neutrophilic: e.g. idiopathic pulmonary fibrosis

Histology
Transbronchial biopsy
Surgical biopsy

Clubbing

Chest X-ray

DIFFUSE PARENCHYMAL
SHADOWING

ALVEOLITIS
(inflammation)

LUNG FIBROSIS
(honeycomb lung)

Organic dusts
Extrinsic allergic alveolitis
e.g. Farmer's lung
     Pigeon fancier's lung
     Budgie fancier's lung

Inorganic dusts
Asbestosis
Coal miner's pneumoconiosis
(see Chapter 15)

Inhaled toxins
Paraquat

Drugs
Amiodarone
Bleomycin
Nitrofurantoin

Systemic diseases
Rheumatoid disease
Systemic sclerosis
Systemic lupus erythematosus
Dermatomyositis
Amyloidosis
Tuberose sclerosis
Neurofibromatosis
Lymphangitis carcinomatosa

Idiopathic
Idiopathic pulmonary fibrosis
Sarcoidosis
Crytogenic organizing pneumonitis

Figure 14.2 Summary of the clinical investigations and differential diagnosis of interstitial lung disease.

of prednisolone and azathioprine but unfortunately the response to treatment is poor and about 50% of patients die within 3 years of diagnosis. For younger patients lung transplantation may be an option (see Chapter 21). More recently the anti-oxidant N-acetylcysteine has been shown to slow the rate of decline in lung function, suggesting that the aberrant fibrosis may involve imbalances in the oxidant—anti-oxidant and protease—anti-protease systems of the lung.

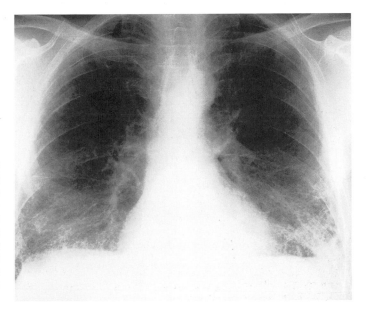

Figure 14.3 This 70-year-old man presented with a 6-month history of progressive breathlessness, crackles and clubbing with reduced lung volumes and impaired gas diffusion. The chest X-ray shows small lung volumes with reticular shadowing particularly affecting the lung peripheries and bases suggesting IPF. He failed to respond to prednisolone and died 1 year later of respiratory failure.

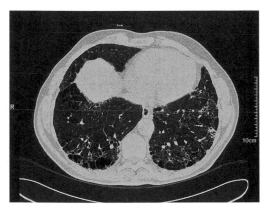

Figure 14.4 HRCT of a 70-year-old man with IPF showing 'honeycombing' which is a cluster or row of cysts due to advanced fibrosis in the subpleural area.

Idiopathic interstitial pneumonias

The broad term 'idiopathic interstitial pneumonias' is used to describe a spectrum of inflammatory and fibrotic lung diseases of unknown cause, including IPF.

Non-specific interstitial pneumonia is characterised by more uniform inflammatory changes and less fibrosis on lung biopsy with correspondingly more ground glass opacification on CT, a better response to corticosteroids and a more favourable prognosis than IPF. In **cryptogenic organising pneumonia** histology shows intra-alveolar buds of organising fibrosis. This seems to be a pattern of response in the lungs to a variety of insults. It particularly occurs in association with some drugs (e.g. amiodarone), connective tissue diseases (e.g. rheumatoid disease) or ulcerative colitis but often no cause is identifiable. Clinically, patients often have cough, malaise, fever, dyspnoea with chest X-ray infiltrates and an elevated erythrocyte sedimentation rate (ESR). Often the patient is thought to have infective pneumonia but the differential diagnosis is widened when no pathogen is identified and the patient fails to respond to antibiotics. There is typically a dramatic response to corticosteroids although relapse may occur as the dose is reduced.

Desquamative interstitial pneumonia and **respiratory bronchiolitis—interstitial lung disease** are relatively rare forms of interstitial lung disease which affect smokers. They have particular features of desquamation of alveolar macrophages or bronchiolitis on biopsy. They respond well to smoking cessation and corticosteroids. **Lymphoid interstitial pneumonia** is characterised by the presence of lymphoid cells in the interstitium. It may occur as a complication of human immunodeficiency virus (HIV) infection or connective

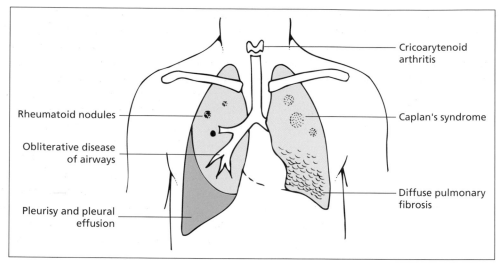

Figure 14.5 Summary of pulmonary complications of rheumatoid disease.

tissue diseases. **Acute interstitial pneumonia** is a very aggressive form of interstitial lung disease characterised by rapidly progressive diffuse alveolar damage.

The idiopathic interstitial pneumonias, therefore, are a complex array of inflammatory and fibrotic lung diseases. The lungs may respond to different insults with a similar pattern of inflammation and fibrosis, and conversely a single agent, such as amiodarone, may produce a range of reactions within the lung. The overall clinical management requires the integration of clinical, radiological and histological features.

Connective tissue diseases

The typical clinical features of IPF with the histopathological pattern of usual interstitial pneumonia can occur in association with a connective tissue disease. These diseases have a number of other lung complications.

Rheumatoid disease (Fig. 14.5)

Involvement of the **crico-arytenoid joint** causes hoarseness and sometimes stridor. **Obliterative bronchiolitis** results in progressive peripheral airways obstruction. **Pleural effusions** are common and analysis of the pleural fluid characteristically

shows a high protein level (exudate) with a low glucose concentration and a high titre of rheumatoid factor. **Rheumatoid nodules** may develop in the lung parenchyma and show the same histological features as the rheumatoid subcutaneous nodules. When rheumatoid disease occurs in association with coalworker's pneumoconiosis, large cavitating pulmonary nodules may develop (**Caplan's syndrome**). Fibrotic lung diseases complicating rheumatoid disease is managed in the same way as IPF, but the prognosis is generally better. Drugs (e.g. methotrexate, infliximab) used to treat rheumatoid disease may cause inflammatory reactions within the lung and may also give rise to lung infections. In these circumstances diffuse infiltrates on chest X-ray could be due to infection, a drug reaction, lung involvement by the connective tissue disease or co-incidental lung disease (see Table 8.3). Bronchoalveolar lavage is useful in detecting infection. Where a drug reaction is suspected information is available on a website (http://www.pneumotox.com) and prompt cessation of the drug and treatment with corticosteroids are important.

Systemic sclerosis (scleroderma)

Diffuse lung fibrosis is the most common complication. **Chest wall restriction** by contraction of the skin is rare. **Aspiration pneumonia** may occur because of oesophageal dysmotility in the CREST variant of the disease: calcinosis, Raynaud's phenomenon, oesophageal dysfunction, sclerodactyly and telangiectasia. **Pulmonary hypertension** may also develop in patients with the CREST syndrome as a primary vascular phenomenon, often in the absence of significant pulmonary fibrosis (see Chapter 16).

Systemic lupus erythematosus

Pleural effusions are common and may cause **pleural thickening**. The phenomenon of 'shrinking lungs', in which the chest X-ray shows high hemidiaphragms with small lungs, is probably caused by myopathy of the diaphragm. Lung fibrosis may occur. Immunosuppressive treatments predispose to **opportunistic infections** (e.g. *Pneumocystis* pneumonia).

Extrinsic allergic alveolitis

Extrinsic allergic alveolitis (hypersensitivity pneumonitis) is an **immunologically mediated lung disease** in which a hypersensitivity response occurs in a **sensitised individual** to an **inhaled antigen**. Typical examples of this disease are **farmer's lung** and **bird fancier's lung**. When hay is harvested and stored in damp conditions it becomes mouldy, generating heat which encourages growth of fungi such as *Thermoactinomyces vulgaris* or *Saacharospora rectivirgula*. When the hay is subsequently used for foddering cattle, fungal spores may be inhaled. Avian antigens are inhaled by people who participate in the sport of pigeon racing or who keep pet birds such as budgerigars. The inhalation of these antigens provokes a complex immune response in susceptible subjects involving antibody reactions, immune-complex formation, complement activation and cellular responses, resulting in alveolitis. Strangely these diseases are less common in smokers.

In the **acute form** of the disease the patient typically experiences recurrent episodes of dyspnoea, dry cough, pyrexia, myalgia and a flu-like sensation, occurring about 4–8 hours after antigen exposure.

During such an episode lung function tests may show a reduction in lung volumes and gas diffusion, and chest X-ray may show diffuse shadowing. Sometimes the chest X-ray may be normal and CT is more sensitive in detecting the changes of extrinsic allergic alveolitis (Fig. 14.6). The acute illness is often misdiagnosed as pneumonia. The **chronic form** is characterised by the insidious development of dyspnoea and lung fibrosis. Lung biopsies show features of fibrosis, alveolitis and granuloma formation. Bronchoalveolar lavage typically shows evidence of a lymphocytic alveolitis with a predominance of T-suppressor lymphocytes. Precipitating antibodies to avian or fungal antigens can be detected in serum but are also found in many asymptomatic subjects so that they are not diagnostic.

Complete **cessation of exposure to the provoking antigen** is the main treatment. However, pigeon fanciers, for example, are very committed to their sport and will often wish to continue keeping pigeons. They can reduce antigen contact by wearing a mask and a loft-coat and hat (so as to avoid carrying antigen on their clothing or hair). **Steroids** (e.g. prednisolone 40 mg/day) hasten the resolution of the alveolitis and are often used during severe acute episodes. The immune response in extrinsic allergic alveolitis is complex and a variety of modulating factors influence the interaction of antigenic stimulus and host response so that the longitudinal course of the disease is variable with some patients developing lung fibrosis and others showing spontaneous improvement despite continued antigen exposure.

Sarcoidosis

Sarcoidosis is a mysterious **multisystem disease** characterised by the occurrence in affected organs of **non-caseating granulomatous lesions** which may progress to cause fibrosis. The aetiology is unknown but the accumulation of CD4 lymphocytes at disease sites is suggestive of an immunological reaction to an unidentified poorly degradable antigen. The frequent involvement of the lungs raises the possibility that such a putative antigen enters the body via the lungs. The

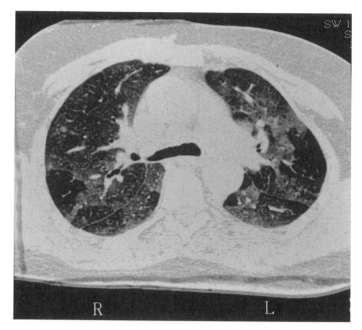

Figure 14.6 This 65-year-old man who kept 150 racing pigeons presented with recurrent episodes of dyspnoea, cough, fever and 'flu'. CT scan shows a characteristic pattern for extrinsic allergic alveolitis of 'ground-glass' shadowing with areas of decreased attenuation and air trapping on expiratory scans.

compartmentalisation of CD4 lymphocytes in affected tissues is associated with a corresponding depletion of CD4 cells in other tissues and depression of some delayed-type hypersensitivity responses such that patients with sarcoidosis often demonstrate negative reactions to tuberculin (i.e. negative Heaf or Mantoux tests despite previous bacillus Calmette–Guérin (BCG) vaccination). Serum immunoglobulin levels are usually elevated and immune complexes are often present in acute sarcoidosis.

The clinical features of sarcoidosis are very varied but it is useful to consider two broad categories of disease: an acute form which is usually transient and often resolves spontaneously; and a chronic form which is persistent and may cause fibrosis (Fig. 14.7).

Acute sarcoidosis

The acute form typically develops abruptly in young adults with **erythema nodosum** and **bilateral hilar lymphadenopathy (BHL)**, sometimes with **uveitis**, **arthritis** and **parotitis**.

Erythema nodosum

This appears as **round red raised nodules**, typically over the shins. It is a manifestation of hypersensitivity and is also found in other diseases such as streptococcal infection, tuberculosis, ulcerative colitis and Crohn's disease, and with drugs (e.g. sulphonamides, contraceptive pill), but in many cases no cause is identified.

Bilateral hilar lymphadenopathy

BHL is not associated with any signs on examination of the chest or with any loss of lung function and is often found incidentally on a **chest X-ray**, but often the X-ray was taken in a patient with other features suggestive of sarcoidosis (Fig. 14.8). Although sarcoidosis is the most common cause of BHL, other causes include lymphoma, metastatic carcinoma, tuberculosis, fungal infections such as coccidioidomycosis and histoplasmosis in endemic areas (e.g. North America); and, in the past, berylliosis (e.g. beryllium used in fluorescent lighting).

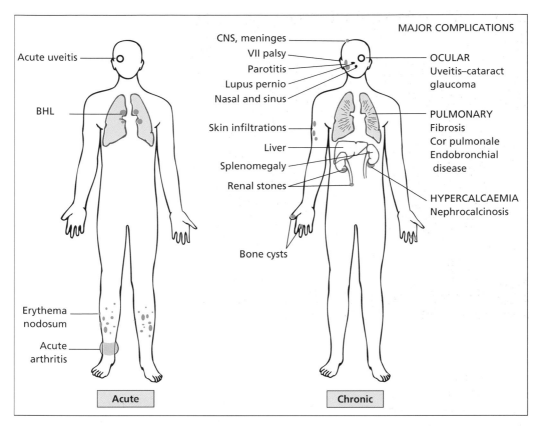

Figure 14.7 Principal clinical features of sarcoidosis.

Chronic sarcoidosis

The chronic form of sarcoidosis pursues a more indolent course, often in an older age group, with involvement of many tissues of the body.

Chronic pulmonary sarcoidosis

This involves the lung parenchyma with **reticular shadowing** often distributed in a perihilar fashion on chest X-ray (Fig. 14.9). There are often remarkably few signs on examination of the chest, and lung function may be well maintained but the disease may progress in some patients causing **progressive fibrosis** and loss of lung function with impairment of gas diffusion, reduction in lung volumes and sometimes airways obstruction with air trapping and bulla formation.

Chronic extrapulmonary sarcoidosis

Sarcoidosis may affect virtually any organ in the body. **Ocular sarcoidosis** often presents as pain and redness of the eye as a result of anterior uveitis. Chorioretinitis, keratoconjunctivitis sicca and lacrimal gland enlargement may complicate chronic sarcoidosis. **Parotid gland enlargement** may be painful and sometimes causes facial nerve palsy. **Central nervous system** involvement may cause cranial nerve palsies, chronic meningitis, obstructive hydrocephalus and a variety of neurological syndromes. **Posterior pituitary** involvement may rarely cause diabetes insipidus. **Cutaneous sarcoidosis** may cause maculopapular eruptions, plaques, nodules and lupus pernio (a violaceous chronic skin lesion particularly affecting the nose and cheeks). **Bone** cysts are sometimes found and

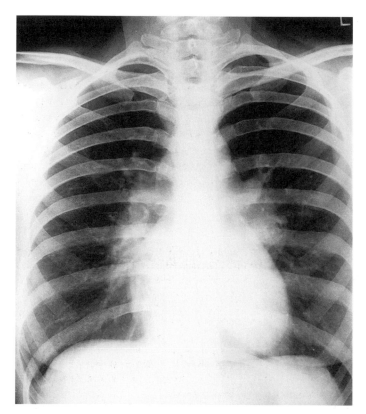

Figure 14.8 This 25-year-old woman presented with uveitis, arthralgia and erythema nodosum of her shins. The chest X-ray shows BHL. She was otherwise well and lung function tests were normal. A diagnosis of probable acute sarcoidosis was made. The disease resolved spontaneously without the need for any medical intervention.

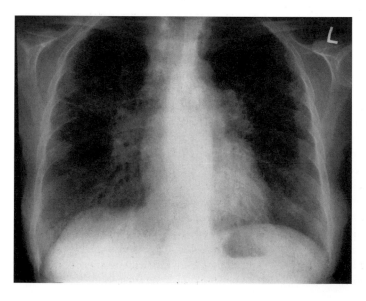

Figure 14.9 This 60-year-old woman presented with cough and progressive breathlessness. There were no crackles on auscultation of her chest but transfer factor for carbon monoxide and transfer coefficient were reduced to 60% of the predicted values. The chest X-ray shows extensive perihilar reticular shadowing. Transbronchial lung biopsy showed non-caseating granulomas and lung fibrosis. Tests for tuberculosis were negative. She was treated with prednisolone with some improvement in lung function.

are often asymptomatic. **Cardiac** sarcoid may cause conduction system damage and arrhythmias. **Hypercalcaemia** may result from increased bone resorption, and nephrocalcinosis, hypercalcuria and renal calculi may occur. Sarcoid granulomas and fibrosis may also be found in the liver, spleen, lymph nodes and muscle, for example.

Diagnosis

The diagnosis of sarcoidosis can often be made on **clinical** grounds, particularly when a young adult presents with classic features such as erythema nodosum and BHL. In less typical cases it is helpful to obtain **biopsy of an affected organ**. **Transbronchial biopsy** is particularly useful and may be combined with **bronchoalveolar lavage**, which typically demonstrates evidence of a CD4 lymphocyte alveolitis. **Mediastinoscopy** and biopsy of hilar lymph nodes is sometimes indicated to exclude other diagnoses such as lymphoma. The histological appearances must be considered in the clinical context because they are not in themselves diagnostic, and other granulomatous disease (e.g. tuberculosis) must be excluded. Serum angiotensin-converting enzyme (ACE) levels are elevated in about two-thirds of patients with active sarcoidosis but this test lacks sensitivity and specificity and is therefore of limited value in diagnosis or in monitoring the course of the disease.

Treatment

In most patients sarcoidosis is a **self-limiting disease** which **resolves spontaneously** without treatment. However, a minority of patients with chronic sarcoidosis develop progressive fibrosis. Because the cause of sarcoidosis is unknown no specific treatment is available but **corticosteroids** suppress inflammation in the affected organs, frequently improving local and systemic symptoms. Their effect on the long-term natural history of sarcoidosis is less clear. They are usually used in patients with progressive disease and studies suggest some benefit from steroid therapy at the cost of adverse effects (e.g. osteoporosis, Cushing's

syndrome). A short course of prednisolone is sometimes used for particularly troublesome acute symptoms such as parotitis, arthritis or erythema nodosum if non-steroidal anti-inflammatory drugs are not sufficient. Uveitis may be treated by topical steroids, and skin manifestations may be amenable to steroid creams or steroid injections. Inhaled steroids have been tried for pulmonary disease but evidence of efficacy is lacking. In chronic sarcoidosis deciding who to treat and when to treat requires **careful judgement to balance the benefit and risks of chronic steroid therapy.**

Keypoints

- Interstitial lung disease typically presents with breathlessness, crackles, reduced gas diffusion and VC and diffuse infiltrates on chest X-ray.
- Exclude other diagnoses, e.g. pulmonary oedema, bronchiectasis, pneumonia, alveolar cell carcinoma.
- Seek potential causes such as drugs (e.g. amiodarone), antigens (e.g. pet birds), occupational dust exposure (e.g. asbestos) and systemic diseases (e.g. rheumatoid disease).
- High-resolution CT shows the pattern and extent of fibrosis and alveolitis and lung biopsy may be needed to determine the histopathological pattern.
- Treatments such as prednisolone and azathioprine should be used judiciously assessing the benefits and adverse effects carefully.

Further reading

American Thoracic Society and European Respiratory Society. Idiopathic pulmonary fibrosis: diagnosis and treatment: international consensus statement. *Am J Respir Crit Care Med* 2000; **161**: 646–64.

American Thoracic Society and European Respiratory Society. International multidisciplinary consensus classification of the idiopathic interstitial pneumonias. *Am J Respir Crit Care Med* 2002; **165**: 277–304.

Bourke SJ, Dalphin JC, Boyd G, McSharry C, Baldwin CI, Calvert JE. Hypersensitivity pneumonitis: current concepts. *Eur Respir J* 2001; **18** (Suppl. 32): 81–92.

British Thoracic Society. The diagnosis, assessment and treatment of diffuse parenchymal lung disease in adults. *Thorax* 1999; **54** (Suppl. 1): 1–30.

Demedts M, Behr J, Buhl R et al. High-dose acetylcysteine in idiopathic pulmonary fibrosis. *N Engl J Med* 2005; **353**: 2229–42.

King TE. Clinical advances in the diagnosis and therapy of interstitial lung diseases. *Am J Respir Crit Care Med* 2005; **172**: 268–79.

Martin W, Iannuzzi MC, Gail DB, Peavy HH. Future directions in sarcoidosis research. *Am J Respir Crit Care Med* 2004; **170**: 567–72.

Pneumotox-drug reactions website. www.pneumotox.com

Westhovens R, DeKeyser F, Van den Hoogen FH et al. The clinical spectrum and pathogenesis of pulmonary manifestations in connective tissue diseases. *Eur Respir Mon* 2006; **34**: 1–26.

Chapter 15

Occupational lung disease

Introduction

The importance of the work environment as a cause of lung disease has been recognised since ancient times. Hippocrates (460–370 BC) taught his pupils to observe the environment of their patients. Ramazzini urged physicians to ask patients what work they did and to visit the workplace. In 1713 he published a treatise on work-related diseases (*De Morbis Artificium*) which included descriptions of baker's asthma and what is now known as extrinsic allergic alveolitis.

Occupational lung diseases result from the inhalation of dusts, gases, fumes or vapours encountered in the workplace, and the hazards of the work environment are constantly changing as old industries are replaced by new ones. The effects of inhaled substances depend on many factors including particle size, physical characteristics (e.g. solubility), toxicity, the intensity and duration of exposures and the person's susceptibility. Particles >10 μm in diameter are usually filtered out of the inhaled airstream in the nose; particles of 1–10 μm are mainly deposited in the bronchi; and particles <1 μm penetrate to the alveoli. Inhaled substances may exert their effects in various ways, and in many circumstances the precise mechanisms involved are incompletely understood. Some substances exert a non-specific **irritant** effect (e.g. generally dusty environment) or are **toxic** to the airways (e.g. chlorine, ammonia) with all workers exposed

being similarly affected. Other substances induce **hypersensitivity** or allergic reactions in susceptible individuals giving rise to asthma or extrinsic allergic alveolitis (see Chapter 14), for example. Some inhaled dusts **promote fibrosis** in the lung parenchyma (e.g. silica, asbestos, coal dust) and some are **carcinogenic** (e.g. cigarette smoke, asbestos). Occasionally, **infective organisms** are inhaled (e.g. *Mycobacterium tuberculosis* in health care workers, *Chlamydia psittaci* in bird handlers). Occupational exposure to **tobacco smoke** is a hazard to those working in places such as bars, restaurants and nightclubs, and smoking bans are being introduced in many places as part of the requirements to provide a safe working environment.

Occupational asthma

Asthma is now the most common type of occupational lung disease. Occupational asthma may be defined as **variable airways obstruction caused by workplace exposures**. In most cases it is due to a **hypersensitivity reaction** to a substance at work but it may result from an **irritant effect** after high exposure to a gas, fume or vapour at work. This definition excludes the triggering of episodes of wheezing in patients with pre-existing asthma by mechanisms such as cold air or exercise at work. Occupational asthma accounts for about 10–15% of cases of asthma in adults. The list of causes of occupational asthma is long and new agents are

Table15.1 Common causes of occupational asthma.

Agent	Occupational exposure
Isocyanates	Spray paints, varnishes, adhesives, polyurethane foam manufacture
Flour	Bakers
Colophony	Electronic soldering flux
Epoxy resins	Hardening agents, adhesives
Animals (rats, mice)	Laboratory workers
Wood dusts	Sawmill workers, joiners
Azodicarbonamide	Polyvinyl plastics manufacture
Persulphate salts	Hairdressers
Latex	Health care workers
Drugs (penicillin, cephalosporins)	Pharmaceutical industry
Grain dust (mites, moulds)	Farmers, millers, bakers

being continuously added. Some of the most common causes are shown in Table 15.1. Occupational asthma is rare amongst library, professional and clerical workers but is common amongst spray painters (isocyanates), bakers (flour), hairdressers (persulphates) and workers in the plastics and chemical industries (epoxy resins, azodicarbonamide), for example.

Diagnosis

To establish a diagnosis of occupational asthma it is first necessary to **confirm the presence of asthma** and, secondly, to show a **causal relationship between the asthma and the work environment**. Although the suspicion of occupational asthma is often based upon the **patient's history**, the diagnosis should be confirmed by **objective tests** wherever possible because of the importance of the diagnosis in terms of managing the patient, identifying the causative agent, reducing the risk to other workers and addressing the medicolegal and compensation aspects of the diagnosis.

Characteristically, there is an initial latent interval of asymptomatic exposure to the agent before symptoms develop. This **latent interval** varies from a few weeks to several years. Once the worker has developed sensitisation to the agent further exposure may provoke an **early asthmatic response** (reaching a peak within 30 minutes), a **late asthmatic response** (occurring 4–12 hours later) or a **dual response**. If an early response occurs, the relationship of symptoms to the work environment is usually apparent. Late responses typically develop the evening after exposure, disturbing sleep and causing cough and wheeze the following morning. Initially, symptoms **improve away from work** on holidays or at weekends and **deteriorate on return to work**. Once asthma becomes established symptoms may persist even when away from the work environment and are also triggered by other factors such as exercise or cold air. Sometimes the sensitising agent also causes rhinitis and dermatitis. Occupational asthma may develop in workers with pre-existing asthma and this may lead to a delay in diagnosis if the relationship of symptoms to the work environment is not recognised. The patient may be exposed to a known inducer of asthma (e.g. paint sprayers using isocyanates) but doctors need to be constantly alert to new causes of occupational asthma. Atopy increases the risk of developing occupational asthma and smoking increases the risk of occupational asthma in workers exposed to isocyanates, for example.

Serial measurement of **peak expiratory flow** or **spirometry** over several days at work and away from work will usually show evidence of variable airways obstruction (the hallmark of asthma) and may demonstrate a relationship between symptoms, airways obstruction and the work environment. Lung function tests may be normal when the patient is seen away from the work environment. Assessment and management of occupational

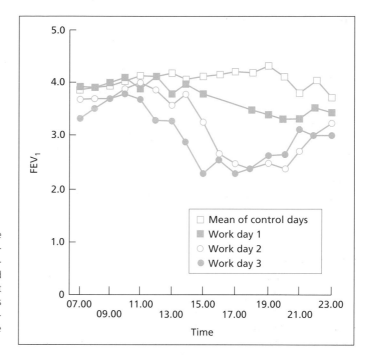

Figure 15.1 Workplace challenge study showing the mean forced expiratory volume in 1 second (FEV$_1$) on control days away from the workplace and progressive falls in FEV$_1$ over 3 days at work indicating late asthmatic reactions of increasing severity occurring in relation to exposure to a biocide in the workplace.

asthma is notoriously difficult as some workers may be reluctant to admit to symptoms in case this jeopardises their employment. Conversely, others may exaggerate symptoms in an attempt to gain compensation. Patients with suspected occupational asthma should therefore be referred for specialist assessment. One of the best ways of showing a relationship between asthma and the work environment is to perform a carefully supervised **workplace challenge study**. In this the patient is removed from the work environment for about 2 weeks and then returned to work under supervision. Serial measurements of spirometry or peak expiratory flow are performed on control days away from work and then over about 3 days on return to the patient's normal work environment. Serial measurements of **airway responsiveness** to methacholine or histamine (see Chapter 11) typically show sequential improvement away from work and rapid deterioration on return to work. Fig. 15.1 shows a typical late asthmatic reaction occurring during a workplace challenge study in a worker in a biocide manufacturing plant. The agent inducing the patient's asthma can often be identified with reasonable confidence by a **visit to the workplace** and an assessment of the materials used. However, workers may be exposed to many agents and it may be difficult to know which agent is causing asthma. **Laboratory challenge studies** involve the patient inhaling the specific suspect agent under double blind, carefully controlled circumstances with serial measurements of spirometry and airway responsiveness. These studies are particularly useful in identifying previously unrecognised causes of occupational asthma but they should only be undertaken in specialist units, as they are potentially hazardous. In some cases of occupational asthma it is possible to demonstrate a positive skin prick test or circulating antibodies to the agent but such immunological reactions are often present in asymptomatic workers also.

Management

Treatment of occupational asthma involves management of both the **affected individual** and the **affected industry**. Early cessation of exposure to the inducing agent may result in complete resolution of the patient's asthma. The key factor in the patient's treatment is therefore not the institution of bronchodilator and steroid treatments as in conventional asthma but the **avoidance of exposure** to the inducing agent. This may be achieved in a number of ways but often involves moving the patient to a different job within the factory. Where there has been a delay in recognising the nature of the patient's asthma and in ceasing exposure chronic asthma may develop which persists even after cessation of contact with the inducing agent, and long-term inhaled steroid and bronchodilator drugs are then required.

Substitution of an alternative non-asthmagenic substance in the industrial process is the ideal solution as this also removes the risk to other workers. Where this is not possible, **enclosure** of the process in a confined booth with **exhaust ventilation** may be possible. **Segregation** of the hazardous process may be useful in limiting the exposure to a small group of workers who are then provided with appropriate personal **protective devices** such as respirator masks. **Surveillance** of other workers should be undertaken where a work environment has been shown to cause asthma. This typically involves a pre-employment medical examination combined with periodic assessment of asthma symptoms, spirometry and, ideally, serial measurements of airway responsiveness. Institution of these measures in the workplace requires the cooperation of the factory safety officer, management, occupational health department and industrial hygienist. Hazards within the workplace fall within the remit of governmental agencies such as the Employment Medical Advisory Service (EMAS) of the Health and Safety Executive in the UK. Workers suffering disability as a result of their employment are entitled to **compensation** from the Department of Social Security in the UK, and may also wish to pursue legal action against their employer where there has been negligence in causing the disease.

Byssinosis

Byssinosis is a particular type of occupational asthma caused by the inhalation of **cotton** or **flax** dust. Symptoms typically arise after several years of working in the industry and show a characteristic pattern different from that seen in typical occupational asthma. Characteristically, workers complain of **chest tightness**, **cough** and **dyspnoea** on Mondays (or the first shift of the week) and, peculiarly, symptoms **improve throughout the working week**. There is sometimes a fall in forced expiratory volume in 1 second (FEV_1) during the working day but there is often a poor correlation between symptoms and FEV_1. Chronic productive cough and irreversible airways obstruction sometimes develop. It is difficult to understand what mechanisms give rise to the pattern of symptoms being worse at the start of the week and improving thereafter. It has been suggested that cotton particles may cause direct release of histamine and that symptoms resolve as histamine stores are depleted. However, the pathogenesis of byssinosis is uncertain, and alternative theories suggest that symptoms may be related to contamination of cotton by Gram-negative bacteria and endotoxins, or that immunological mechanisms may be important.

Popcorn worker's lung

Recently cases of severe **obliterative bronchiolitis** have been reported in workers in popcorn production plants due to inhalation of diacetyl, a ketone with butter-flavour characteristics. The patients developed progressive cough, breathlessness and wheeze with fixed airways obstruction. Computed tomography (CT) scans showed bronchial wall thickening and air trapping, and lung biopsies showed inflammation and occlusion of the small airways in the form of obliterative bronchiolitis. Doctors need to be vigilant in order to detect new causes of occupational lung disease.

Pneumoconiosis

Pneumoconiosis is a general term used to describe lung fibrosis resulting from inhalation of dusts such as coal, silica or asbestos.

Coalworker's pneumoconiosis

The development of pneumoconiosis is directly related to the total exposure to coal dust. Dust exposure varies in different parts of the coalmine and is heaviest at the coalface. Improvements in

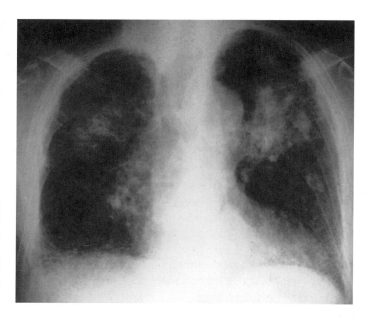

Figure 15.2 This 78-year-old man, who had been a faceworker in a coalmine for 40 years, presented with progressive breathlessness. Chest X-ray shows irregular opacities of progressive massive fibrosis in both upper lobes with extensive background nodular shadowing of coalworker's pneumoconiosis.

ventilation and working conditions have considerably reduced the level of dust in modern coalmines. In many countries there has been a decline in the coal industry with increased use of alternative sources of energy. Coal dust inhaled into the alveoli is taken up by macrophages which are then cleared via the lymphatic drainage system or via the mucociliary escalator of the bronchial tree. If there is heavy prolonged exposure to dust the clearance mechanisms are overwhelmed and dust macules arise particularly in the region of the respiratory bronchioles. Release of dust from dying macrophages induces fibroblast proliferation and fibrosis. There is an important distinction to be made between the two major categories of coalworker's pneumoconiosis.

• *Simple coalworker's pneumoconiosis*: It consists of the accumulation, within the lung tissue, of small (<5 mm) aggregations of coal particles which are uniformly dispersed and evident on chest X-ray as a delicate micronodular mottling. **Simple pneumoconiosis is not associated with any significant symptoms, signs, impairment of lung function or alteration to prognosis, for example life expectancy.** The size and extent of the nodules can be categorised for research and classification purposes by comparing the patient's X-ray with standard films published by the International Labour Office. The benign nature of simple pneumoconiosis is sometimes not appreciated and there is often a tendency to attribute any respiratory symptoms to the pneumoconiosis, whereas alternative explanations such as chronic obstructive pulmonary disease (COPD), asthma or heart disease are more likely to account for the patient's symptoms.

• *Complicated coalworker's pneumoconiosis* (progressive massive fibrosis): It is characterised by the occurrence of large black fibrotic masses in the lung parenchyma, consisting of coal dust and bundles of collagen. These are typically situated in the upper zones and appear as rather **bizarre opacities on chest X-ray** against the background of simple pneumoconiosis (Fig. 15.2). **Cavitation** of these lesions may occur and may result in the expectoration of black sputum (melanoptysis). Complicated pneumoconiosis often results in dyspnoea, a **restrictive ventilatory defect** (reduced lung volumes) and **impaired gas diffusion** (reduced transfer factor for carbon monoxide), and **reduced life expectancy.**

Caplan's syndrome (rheumatoid pneumoconiosis)

Coalworkers with **rheumatoid arthritis** may develop **multiple nodules** of about 0.5–2 cm in diameter in the lungs. These lung nodules are often accompanied by the occurrence of subcutaneous rheumatoid nodules.

Coalworker's bronchitis and emphysema

Coalminers have a high prevalence of **bronchitis**, **airways obstruction** and **emphysema** and since 1993 they have been eligible for compensation from the Department of Social Security in the UK if they have worked underground in coal mines for at least 20 years and have reduced FEV_1.

Silicosis

This is a form of pneumoconiosis resulting from the inhalation of free silica (silicon dioxide). It is now uncommon in developed countries because of widespread recognition and control of the hazards of respirable silica dust, but it still occurs in developing countries. There is a risk of silicosis in workers involved in: **quarrying**, grinding and dressing of sandstone, granite and slate; developing **tunnels** and sinking shafts (e.g. coalmines); **boiler scaling**; **sandblasting** of castings in iron and steel foundries; and the **pottery** industry where silica may be used in the lining of kilns and the dry-grinding of ceramic products.

Simple nodular silicosis, like simple coalworker's pneumoconiosis, causes no symptoms and is an X-ray phenomenon. Complicated silicosis, however, results in **progressive fibrosis**, loss of lung function and dyspnoea. The silicotic nodule consists of concentric layers of collagen surrounding a central area of dust including quartz crystals and dying macrophages. There is a significantly increased risk of **tuberculosis** in patients with silicosis as silica interferes with the ability of macrophages to kill tubercle bacilli. Patients with silicosis are also at increased risk of developing **lung cancer**.

A chest X-ray typically shows **nodular opacities** particularly affecting the **upper lobes**. The nodules are usually denser and larger than those seen in simple coalworker's pneumoconiosis. **Eggshell calcification** of **hilar lymph nodes** is a particularly characteristic feature (Fig. 15.3). **Pleural thickening** may also occur.

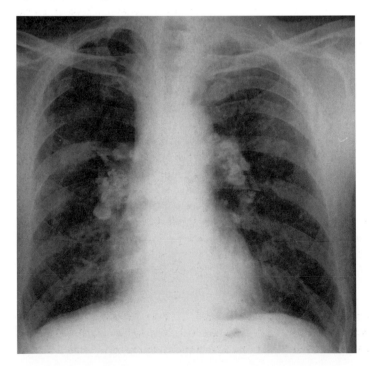

Figure 15.3 This 65-year-old man had had extensive exposure to silica when working in a stone quarry. Chest X-ray shows eggshell calcification (a rim of calcification around the outer margin) of the hilar lymph nodes with upper lobe fibrosis. Tests for tuberculosis were negative.

Siderosis

Dust containing **iron** and its oxides is encountered at various stages in the iron and steel industry and in welding. It gives rise to a simple pneumoconiosis (siderosis) which produces a striking mottled appearance on the chest X-ray because of the high radiodensity of iron, but which is not accompanied by symptoms, signs or any physiological defect. Other metals such as antimony and tin may produce a similar picture.

Asbestos-related lung disease

Asbestos is a collective term for a number of naturally occurring fibrous mineral silicates which are widely used because of their fire-resistant and insulation properties. Asbestos fibres are of two main types which have different physical and chemical properties: *serpentine asbestos fibres* (**chrysotile—white asbestos**) are wispy, flexible and relatively long, such that they are less easily inhaled to the periphery of the lung; *amphibole asbestos fibres* (e.g. **crocidolite—blue asbestos, amosite—brown asbestos, tremolite**) are straighter, stiffer and more brittle, and penetrate more deeply into the lung. They are also more resistant to breakdown within the lung.

Workers may be exposed to asbestos in many different settings so that it is important to take a detailed history of all the patient's occupations over the years and of the tasks undertaken. **Pipe laggers** and industrial **plumbers** often have had heavy exposure to asbestos because it is widely used for **thermal insulation** in **ships**, **power stations** and factories. Many workers in the **shipbuilding** industry were heavily exposed to asbestos when they worked alongside pipe laggers in confined spaces such as the engine rooms of ships. Sometimes housewives washing their husbands' work overalls inhaled significant amounts of asbestos. Workers in the **insulation industry** and those producing **asbestos products** may have been heavily exposed. Chrysotile asbestos is used in **brake-pad linings**, in **cement products**, in **pipes**, **tiles** and **roofing** materials. In many circumstances the asbestos is safely bound within composite materials but respirable dust may be produced by the **cutting of asbestos sheets**, or in demolition work involving the removal, or **stripping-off**, of asbestos insulation from pipes or boilers.

Strict precautions were eventually widely introduced in the 1970s to restrict exposure to asbestos with the use of protective respirators and exhaust ventilation, and the substitution of other materials where possible. However, the long lag interval between the inhalation of asbestos and the development of disease means that asbestos-related lung disease is still all too common. There are several different diseases related to asbestos exposure (Fig. 15.4) and they each have very different manifestations and prognosis.

• *Asbestosis*: Asbestosis is a pneumoconiosis in which **diffuse parenchymal lung fibrosis** develops as a result of heavy prolonged exposure to asbestos. The lag interval between exposure and the onset of the disease is typically 10–25 years, and is shorter the more intense the exposure. The clinical features are similar to those of other interstitial lung diseases such as idiopathic pulmonary fibrosis, with **cough**, progressive **dyspnoea**, bibasal **crackles**, frequently **clubbing** and a **restrictive ventilatory defect** (reduced lung volumes) with **impaired gas diffusion** (reduced transfer factor for carbon monoxide). Chest X-ray shows bilateral **reticulonodular shadowing**. CT is more sensitive in detecting early changes. Fibrosis is usually first evident around the respiratory bronchioles at the lung bases, becoming more diffuse as the disease progresses. **Asbestos bodies**, consisting of an asbestos fibre coated with an iron-containing protein, are usually seen within areas of fibrosis on light or electron microscopy. The disease is usually slowly progressive even after exposure has ceased, and is not usually responsive to corticosteroids. Patients with asbestosis are at substantial risk of developing lung cancer. It seems likely that some individuals have an increased susceptibility to developing asbestosis, although the nature of this susceptibility is unknown.

• *Pleural plaques*: Pleural plaques are often visible as an incidental finding on chest X-rays of workers who have been exposed to asbestos. They are often calcified and appear as **dense white lines** on

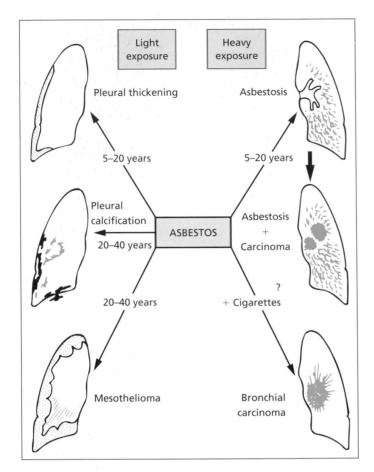

Figure 15.4 Pulmonary diseases relating to exposure to asbestos.

the pleura of the chest wall, diaphragm, pericardium and mediastinum. When seen face-on they form an irregular 'holly leaf' pattern (Fig. 15.5). They consist of white fibrous tissue usually situated on the parietal pleura. They do not give rise to any impairment of lung function or disability.

• *Asbestos pleurisy and pleural effusions*: Many years after first exposure to asbestos, patients may develop episodes of pleurisy with pleuritic pain and pleural effusions. The pleural fluid is an exudate which is often bloodstained even in the absence of malignancy. There is sometimes associated elevation of erythrocyte sedimentation rate (ESR). Other causes of pleural effusion need to be excluded. Pleural biopsy shows evidence of inflammation and fibrosis without any specific diagnostic features. There is usually spontaneous resolution but

recurrent episodes affecting both sides may occur and may lead to pleural thickening.

• *Pleural thickening*: Localised or diffuse thickening and fibrosis of the pleura may develop as a result of asbestos exposure. There may be a history of recurrent episodes of acute pleurisy although these are often subclinical. The pleural thickening is usually most marked at the lung bases with obliteration of the costophrenic angles. It may initially be unilateral but often becomes bilateral. Areas of fibrous strands extending from the thickened pleura may give the appearance of 'crow's feet' on X-ray and rolled atelectasis may appear as a rounded opacity caused by puckering of the lung by the thickened pleura. When the pleural thickening is extensive it causes dyspnoea and a restrictive ventilatory defect.

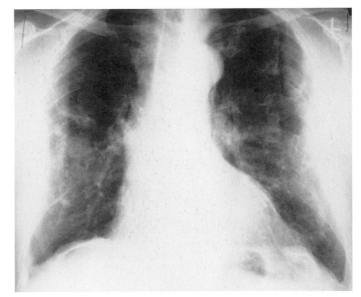

Figure 15.5 This 70-year-old man had had extensive exposure to asbestos when he worked as a pipe lagger in shipyards. His chest X-ray shows extensive calcified pleural plaques seen as dense white lines over the diaphragm and pericardium, and demonstrating a 'holly leaf' pattern when seen face-on over the mid zones of the lungs. There is pleural thickening in both mid zones with some blunting of the costophrenic angles.

- *Asbestos-related lung cancer*: Epidemiology studies show an increased risk of lung cancer in workers in the asbestos industry with an approximately linear relationship between the dose of asbestos and the occurrence of lung cancer. The interaction between **asbestos** and **smoking** is multiplicative. The clinical features, distribution of cell type, investigation and treatment of asbestos-related lung cancers are the same as for those not associated with asbestos exposure (see Chapter 13) but impairment of lung function as a result of asbestosis may preclude surgery. At present, in the UK, workers are entitled to compensation from the Department of Social Security for asbestos-related lung cancer only if it occurs in association with asbestosis or diffuse pleural thickening.

- *Mesothelioma*: It is a **malignant tumour of the pleura** which is associated with a history of asbestos exposure in at least 90% of cases. The risk is greatest in those exposed to **crocidolite (blue asbestos)**. Sometimes the period of exposure to asbestos may have been as short as a few months. At present there are about 2000 deaths each year in the UK from mesothelioma and the incidence is expected to continue to rise until about the year 2020 because effective controls on asbestos exposure were only widely introduced in the 1970s and there is an average **lag interval of 20–40 years** between exposure to asbestos and the development of mesothelioma. It usually presents with **pain, dyspnoea, weight loss and lethargy**, and features of a **pleural effusion** sometimes associated with a lobulated pleural mass on X-ray (Fig. 15.6). **CT scan** typically shows nodular pleural thickening encasing the lung and involving the mediastinal pleura. Video assisted thoracoscopic **pleural biopsy** may be needed for definitive histopathological diagnosis and pleurodesis can be performed at the same time for control of a pleural effusion. As the tumour progresses it encases the lung and may involve the pericardium and peritoneum, and give rise to blood-borne metastases. Radical surgery in the form of **extrapleural pneumonectomy** can be attempted in only a small percentage of patients and has a poor success rate. **Radiotherapy** can reduce the risk of spread of the tumour through biopsy tracks and may relieve pain. **Chemotherapy**, using drugs such as pemetrexed and cisplatin, results in tumour shrinkage in about 40% of patients, with a small improvement in survival rates. Unfortunately prognosis is poor, with most patients **dying within 2 years** of diagnosis.

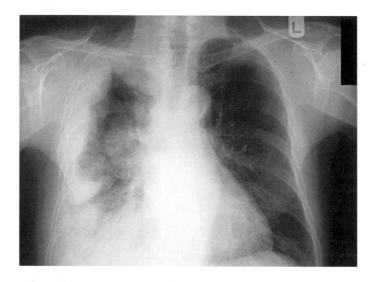

Figure 15.6 This 74-year-old man presented with right sided chest pain and progressive breathlessness. He had been exposed to asbestos 40 years previously in his job as a plumber. His chest X-ray shows extensive lobulated pleural masses encasing the right lung. Percutaneous pleural biopsy showed malignant mesothelioma.

Patients who have suffered disability as a result of occupational lung disease have a statutory right to receive **compensation** from governmental agencies such as the Department of Social Security in the UK. In some cases they may wish to pursue **litigation** against their employer. The death of a patient with a suspected occupational lung disease should be reported to the relevant authority, such as the **coroner**, who may wish to undertake a **post-mortem examination**.

Keypoints

- Asthma is the commonest type of occupational lung disease.
- Occupational asthma accounts for 10–15% of all cases of asthma in adults.
- Avoidance of exposure to the inducing agent is the main treatment of occupational asthma.
- Pneumoconiosis is a form of lung fibrosis due to inhalation of dusts such as asbestos, coal and silica.
- Mesothelioma is a malignant tumour of the pleura due to inhalation of asbestos 20–40 years previously.

Further reading

Akpinar-Elci M, Travis WD, Lynch DA, Kreiss K. Bronchiolitis obliterans in popcorn production plant workers. *Eur Respir J* 2004; **24**: 298–302.

British Lung Foundation: Information on Asbestos and Mesothelioma: www.lunguk.org

British Thoracic Society. Statement on malignant mesothelioma in the United Kingdom. *Thorax* 2001; **56**: 250–65.

Edwards PR, Van Tongeren M, Watson A, Gee I, Edwards RE. Environmental tobacco smoke. *Occup Environ Med* 2004; **61**: 385–6.

McDonald JC, Chen Y, Zekveld C, Cherry NM. Incidence by occupation and industry of acute work related respiratory diseases in the UK, 1992–2001. *Occup Environ Med* 2005; **62**: 836–42.

Nicholson PJ, Cullinan P, Newman Taylor AJ, Burge PS, Boyle C. Evidence based guidelines for the prevention, identification, and management of occupational asthma. *Occup Environ Med* 2005; **62**: 290–9.

Soutar CA, Hurley JF, Miller BG, Cowie HA, Buchanan D. Dust concentrations and respiratory risks in coalminers. *Occup Environ Med* 2004; **61**: 477–81.

Vogelzang NJ, Rusthoven JJ, Symanowski J et al. Phase III study of pemetrexed in combination with cisplatin versus cisplatin alone in patients with malignant pleural mesothelioma. *J Clin Oncol* 2003; **21**: 2636–44.

Chapter 16

Pulmonary vascular disease

Pulmonary embolism

It is estimated that pulmonary emboli occur in about 1% of patients admitted to hospital and are directly responsible for about 5% of all deaths in hospital. The thrombus typically develops in the deep veins of the legs and then travels to the lungs causing obstruction of the pulmonary vasculature. Patients who are immobilised in the community or in hospital are particularly vulnerable to developing deep vein thrombosis (DVT) and then pulmonary embolism. It is the commonest cause of death after elective surgery and is the commonest cause of maternal death in the UK. Strategies to defend against this killer rely on widespread use of subcutaneous heparin prophylaxis against DVT and rapid resort to full anti-coagulation pending definitive investigations, in patients showing features suggesting DVT or pulmonary embolism.

Deep vein thrombosis

Factors predisposing to venous thrombosis were described by Virchow as a triad of venous stasis, damage to the wall of the vein and hypercoagulable states:

- *Venous stasis* occurs as a result of **immobility** (e.g. bed-bound patients on medical, surgical or obstetric wards, airplane flights), **local pressure** (e.g. tight plaster of Paris), **venous obstruction** (e.g. pressure of a pelvic tumour, pregnancy, obesity,

varicose veins), congestive **cardiac failure** and **dehydration**.
- *Damage to a vein* occurs from local **trauma** to the vein, **previous thrombosis** and **inflammation** (phlebitis).
- *Hypercoagulable states* arise as part of the body's response to **surgery**, **trauma** and **childbirth**, and are found in association with **malignancy** and use of **oral oestrogen contraceptives**. Recurrent thrombosis is particularly likely to occur where there are specific heredited abnormalities of the clotting system such as **factor V Leiden gene mutation**, **anti-thrombin III**, **protein S** or **protein C deficiencies** and in **anti-cardiolipin antibody** disease. Patients with recurrent or unexplained thromboembolic disease should have specific tests for these conditions because long-term anti-coagulation is advisable.

Pulmonary embolism is particularly common when thrombosis occurs in the proximal femoral or iliac veins and is less likely to occur when thrombosis is confined to the calf veins. Most pulmonary emboli arise in the deep veins of the legs but they may occasionally arise from thrombus in the inferior vena cava, the right side of the heart or from indwelling catheters in the subclavian or jugular veins. DVT may cause permanent damage to the vein with impairment of venous drainage, oedema, pigmentation, ulceration and an increased risk of further thrombosis.

The classic signs of DVT are oedema of the leg with tenderness, erythema and pain on flexing the ankle (Homan's sign). However, thrombosis in the deep veins of the leg, pelvis or abdomen may be completely silent. DVT must be distinguished from other conditions such as cellulitis, muscle injury or ruptured cysts of the knee and **compression ultrasound** of the leg veins is the usual investigation used to confirm or exclude the diagnosis. Other investigations for detecting DVT include **venography** whereby injection of radiocontrast material outlines thrombus and ^{125}**I-fibrinogen isotope scan** which demonstrates incorporation of radiolabelled fibrinogen into the thrombus.

Clinical features

The clinical features of pulmonary embolism depend upon the size and severity of the embolism, as summarised in Fig. 16.1, although there is overlap between the different presentations. In **acute massive pulmonary embolism** the picture is often that of a patient recovering from recent surgery who collapses. Attempts at resuscitation are often unsuccessful and there is a rapid high mortality, with very limited opportunity for intervention. Occlusion of a large part of the pulmonary circulation produces a catastrophic drop in cardiac output and the patient collapses with hypotension, cyanosis, tachypnoea and engorged neck veins. Sometimes the presentation is more **subacute**, as a series of emboli progressively occlude the pulmonary circulation over a longer period of time, with the patient developing progressive dyspnoea, tachypnoea and hypoxaemia. **Acute minor pulmonary embolism** presents as dyspnoea, typically accompanied by pleuritic pain, haemoptysis and fever if there is associated **pulmonary infarction**. Prompt recognition and treatment of an acute minor embolism may prevent the occurrence of a massive embolism. **Chronic thromboembolic pulmonary hypertension** is an unusual condition in which recurrent emboli progressively occlude the pulmonary circulation giving rise to progressive dyspnoea, pulmonary hypertension and right heart failure.

Pulmonary embolism is both under- and over-diagnosed in clinical practice leading to some patients failing to receive treatment for a potentially life-threatening condition and others being subjected to the risks of anti-coagulant therapy unnecessarily. While it is crucial to confirm a clinical suspicion of pulmonary embolism by a definitive test, it is also important to avoid subjecting large numbers of patients to unnecessary and expensive investigations. Dyspnoea, tachypnoea (respiratory rate >20/min) and pleuritic pain are the three cardinal features of pulmonary embolism. The absence of any of these clinical features makes a diagnosis of pulmonary embolism very unlikely.

Investigations

General investigations

General investigations may yield clues that point towards a diagnosis of pulmonary embolism and are particularly useful in excluding alternative diagnoses:

- *Chest X-ray* is often normal but **elevation of a hemidiaphragm** and areas of **linear atelectasis** are suggestive of pulmonary emboli. A small **pleural effusion** with **wedge-shaped peripheral opacities** may occur in association with pulmonary infarction, and rarely an area of lung infarction undergoes cavitation. In massive embolism an **area of underperfusion** with few vascular markings may be apparent. **Enlarged pulmonary** arteries are a feature of pulmonary hypertension in chronic thromboembolic disease. The chest X-ray helps exclude alternative diagnoses such as pneumothorax, pneumonia and pulmonary oedema.
- *Electrocardiogram* (ECG) is often normal apart from showing a **sinus tachycardia**. In major pulmonary embolism there may be features of **right heart strain** with depression of the ST segment and T wave in leads V_1–V_3, and evidence of right axis deviation with an **S1 Q3 T3** pattern. The ECG helps exclude myocardial infarction and cardiac arrhythmias.
- *Arterial blood gases*: Characteristically pulmonary embolism is associated with ventilation of underperfused areas of lung resulting in hypoxaemia

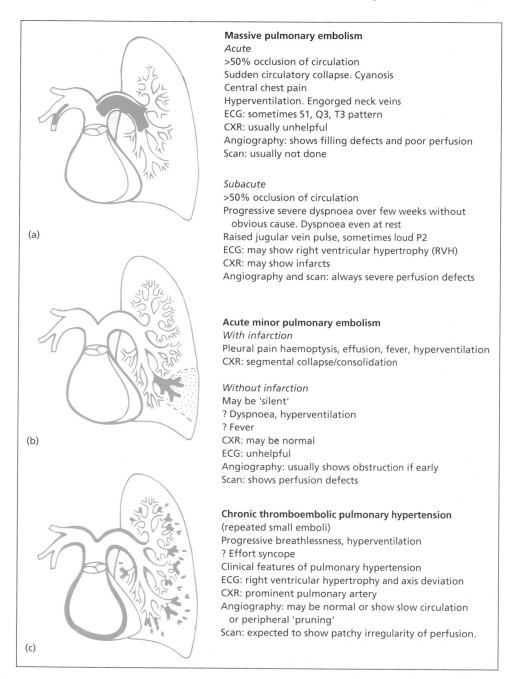

Massive pulmonary embolism
Acute
>50% occlusion of circulation
Sudden circulatory collapse. Cyanosis
Central chest pain
Hyperventilation. Engorged neck veins
ECG: sometimes S1, Q3, T3 pattern
CXR: usually unhelpful
Angiography: shows filling defects and poor perfusion
Scan: usually not done

Subacute
>50% occlusion of circulation
Progressive severe dyspnoea over few weeks without
  obvious cause. Dyspnoea even at rest
Raised jugular vein pulse, sometimes loud P2
ECG: may show right ventricular hypertrophy (RVH)
CXR: may show infarcts
Angiography and scan: always severe perfusion defects

Acute minor pulmonary embolism
With infarction
Pleural pain haemoptysis, effusion, fever, hyperventilation
CXR: segmental collapse/consolidation

Without infarction
May be 'silent'
? Dyspnoea, hyperventilation
? Fever
CXR: may be normal
ECG: unhelpful
Angiography: usually shows obstruction if early
Scan: shows perfusion defects

Chronic thromboembolic pulmonary hypertension
(repeated small emboli)
Progressive breathlessness, hyperventilation
? Effort syncope
Clinical features of pulmonary hypertension
ECG: right ventricular hypertrophy and axis deviation
CXR: prominent pulmonary artery
Angiography: may be normal or show slow circulation
  or peripheral 'pruning'
Scan: expected to show patchy irregularity of perfusion.

Figure 16.1 Synopsis of pulmonary embolism.

and hyperventilation so that arterial blood gases show a reduced P_{O_2} and P_{CO_2}.
• *Lung function tests* are not usually helpful in the acute situation but in patients with dyspnoea caused by chronic or subacute pulmonary emboli there is reduced gas diffusion with a reduction in the transfer factor for carbon monoxide. Lung function tests may also help identify other lung diseases

(e.g. chronic obstructive pulmonary disease (COPD) and emphysema).

- *Blood tests*: There may be evidence of intravascular thrombosis (thrombin–anti-thrombin III complex assay) and fibrinolysis (fibrin degradation products). D-**dimer** is a breakdown product of cross-linked fibrin and levels are elevated in patients with thromboembolism. However, levels are also often elevated in other hospitalised patients so that D-dimer assays can be used to exclude, but not to confirm venous thromboembolism. A normal D-dimer level can be particularly useful in certain clinical settings. For example, a young woman on oral contraception who presents with isolated pleuritic pain is very unlikely to have pulmonary embolism if the respiratory rate is below 20/min and chest X-ray, arterial blood gases and D-dimer are normal. She can be reassured without the need for admission to hospital or further investigation.

Specific investigations

- *Pulmonary angiography* is the definitive test for diagnosing pulmonary embolism but it is an invasive test requiring specialist expertise and equipment which are not widely available, and it is associated with a small risk, particularly in critically ill patients. A catheter is passed from a peripheral vein (e.g. femoral vein), through the right side of the heart into the pulmonary arteries, and radiocontrast material is injected and a rapid sequence of X-rays is taken. The angiographic features of embolism are intraluminal filling defects, abrupt cut-off of vessels, peripheral pruning of vessels and areas of reduced perfusion.

Computed tomography pulmonary angiography **(CTPA)** (Fig. 16.2) is increasingly being used as the definitive initial non-invasive imaging modality for pulmonary embolism. Very rapid spiral images are obtained during the injection of iodinated contrast medium into a peripheral vein. It has better specificity than ventilation–perfusion isotope scanning in the diagnosis of pulmonary embolism although it does involve a higher radiation dose. It also provides information on a potential alternative diagnosis when pulmonary embolism is excluded:

- *Ventilation/perfusion (V/Q) lung scan*: Macro-aggregated particles or microspheres of human albumin, labelled with a gamma-emitting radioisotope, technetium-99m, are injected intravenously. These particles impact in the pulmonary capillaries and the radioactivity emitted from the lung fields is detected by a gamma camera, thus outlining the distribution of pulmonary perfusion. The distribution of ventilation in the lungs is similarly

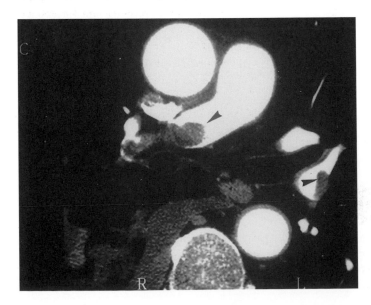

Figure 16.2 Computed tomography (CT) pulmonary angiogram showing clot in the main pulmonary artery of the right lung (upper arrow) and the lower lobe pulmonary artery of the left lung (lower arrow).

outlined after the patient has inhaled radiolabelled xenon. A completely normal pattern of pulmonary perfusion is strong evidence against pulmonary embolism. 'Cold areas' are evident on the scan where there is defective blood flow and these may occur in association with localised abnormalities apparent on a chest X-ray (e.g. pleural effusion, carcinoma, bulla). In these circumstances ventilation is usually decreased in the same areas resulting in 'matched defects' in ventilation and perfusion scans. The classic pattern seen in pulmonary embolism consists of multiple areas of perfusion defects that are not matched with defects in ventilation. A *V/Q* scan may therefore show normal perfusion, in which case pulmonary embolism is unlikely ('low probability'), areas of perfusion defects not matched with ventilation defects in the presence of a normal chest X-ray which indicates a 'high probability' of pulmonary embolism, or it may show matched ventilation and perfusion defects in which case interpretation is difficult and the scan is regarded as 'indeterminate'. Patients with a suspected pulmonary embolism but an indeterminate scan require further imaging:

• *Imaging of peripheral veins*: Demonstration of thrombus in the peripheral veins by venography, Doppler ultrasound or ^{125}I-fibrinogen isotope scan provides support for the decision to anti-coagulate a patient who has clinical features of pulmonary embolism but an 'indeterminate' *V/Q* scan.

Diagnosing pulmonary embolism

The diagnosis or exclusion of pulmonary embolism involves a careful clinical assessment through a series of steps:

• **Clinical features compatible** with pulmonary embolism are present, notably breathlessness or increased respiratory rate with or without pleuritic pain or haemoptysis.

• **Alternative diagnoses** (e.g. pneumothorax, pneumonia) are excluded.

• **Risk factors** are assessed to determine the likelihood of venous thromboembolic disease.

• D-**dimer level** is measured. A negative D-dimer assay has an important role in accurately excluding venous thromboembolic disease.

• Definitive imaging (e.g. **CTPA** or V/Q scanning) is performed.

Treatment

Anti-coagulant therapy

When a clinical diagnosis of suspected pulmonary embolism or DVT has been made, anti-coagulants should be started at once unless there is a strong contraindication (e.g. active haemorrhage). The decision as to whether anti-coagulants should be continued in the long term is made later based upon the results of subsequent investigations. **Low-molecular weight heparin** (e.g. **tinzaparin** 175 units/kg subcutaneously once daily) is now the standard initial treatment for patients with pulmonary embolism. The dose is determined by the patient's weight and anti-coagulant monitoring is not needed. An alternative is unfractionated heparin (e.g. heparin given as an initial intravenous bolus followed by an infusion), and this requires monitoring of the activated partial thromboplastin time (APPT) with adjustment of the dose to maintain the APPT at 1.5–2.5 times the control value. Intravenous heparin may be preferred to subcutaneous heparin in patients with a massive pulmonary embolism or where rapid reversal of anti-coagulation may be needed (e.g. in patients at risk of haemorrhage). Side-effects of heparin include haemorrhage, bruising and thrombocytopenia. Once the clinical suspicion of pulmonary embolism or DVT has been supported by subsequent investigations **oral anti-coagulation** is commenced using **warfarin**. Usually, 10 mg is given on the first day as a loading dose, and then the international normalised ratio (INR) is measured and the dosage adjusted to maintain a ratio of about 2–3. Warfarin takes at least 48–72 hours to establish its anti-coagulant effect so that heparin needs to be continued for this period. The optimal duration of warfarin treatment is uncertain but it is usually continued for 3–6 months after a first episode of idiopathic venous thromboembolism. Patients with recurrent or unexplained thromboembolic disease should have investigations for hypercoagulable states performed (e.g. anti-thrombin III, protein S or C deficiencies; anti-cardiolipin antibody disease) and may require long-term anti-coagulation.

The patient should be given an **anti-coagulant information booklet** which explains the nature and side-effects of treatment, states the indication for and proposed duration of treatment, contact numbers for obtaining advice and instructions on avoiding medications which interfere with therapy. Many drugs enhance the effect of warfarin (e.g. non-steroidal anti-inflammatory drugs, aspirin, ciprofloxacin, erythromycin, etc.) and others reduce the effect (e.g. carbamazepine, barbiturates, rifampicin, etc.). Warfarin is teratogenic and women of child-bearing age should be warned of this danger, and may require specialist contraceptive advice. Precise details of INR, warfarin dosage and clinic appointments are included in the booklet which provides a useful method of communication with the patient and with all involved in the care of the patient (e.g. general practitioner, dentist, nurses, etc.).

Thrombolytic therapy

The aim of thrombolytic therapy is to actively dissolve clot, but its use is reserved for those patients with acute massive pulmonary embolism who remain in severe haemodynamic collapse (e.g. hypotensive, poorly perfused, hypoxaemic). These patients have survived the immediate impact of the pulmonary embolism but remain critically ill. If all the clinical features and bedside tests (e.g. ECG, chest X-ray) suggest a massive pulmonary embolism and exclude alternative diagnoses (pneumothorax, post-operative haemorrhage, etc.), a decision may have to be taken that the circumstances justify the use of thrombolytic therapy. Contraindications to thrombolytic therapy include active haemorrhage, recent major surgery or trauma. Typically alteplase 50 mg is given as a bolus via a peripheral vein. Thereafter heparin anti-coagulation is commenced.

Patients with acute pulmonary embolism require **high-flow oxygen** to correct hypoxaemia, and **analgesia** (e.g. diamorphine) to relieve pain and distress. In patients with active haemorrhage contraindicating the use of anti-coagulant, or recurrent pulmonary emboli despite adequate

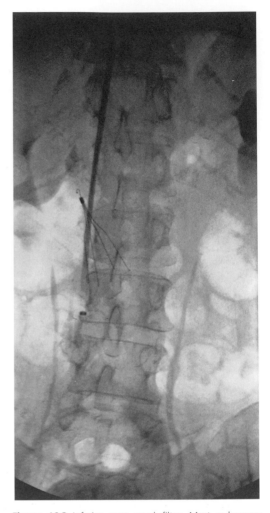

Figure 16.3 Inferior vena caval filter. Most pulmonary emboli arise from thrombi in the deep veins of the leg. An inferior vena caval filter can be used to prevent emboli from reaching the lungs. They are used in patients who have suffered recurrent pulmonary emboli despite adequate anti-coagulation and in those in whom anti-coagulant therapy is contraindicated. This 64-year-old woman had had major pulmonary emboli from a DVT in her right femoral vein. She then suffered major haemorrhage from a gastric ulcer while on heparin therapy, which was discontinued. A filter device was passed through the venous system from the internal jugular vein to be placed in the inferior vena cava.

anti-coagulation, **a venous filter** procedure may be useful. This involves the passing of a specially designed filter into the inferior vena cava to prevent further emboli from reaching the lungs from DVT in the pelvis or lower limbs (Fig. 16.3).

DVT prophylaxis

A variety of measures are directed against Virchow's triad of factors predisposing to DVT. Early **ambulation**, use of graded elastic **compression stockings** and leg **exercises** reduce venous stasis. Prophylactic **low-dose heparin** is now widely used to reduce the risk for patients on surgical, obstetric and medical wards. Typically, tinzaparin 3500 units/day is given subcutaneously. For patients undergoing surgery with a higher risk of DVT (e.g. hip replacement) the dosage may be increased to 4500 units given 12 hours before surgery and then daily until the patient is mobile again.

Other materials which may occasionally embolise to the lungs include **fat** (after fracture of long bones), **amniotic fluid** (post-partum), **air** (e.g. from disconnected central venous lines), **tumour** (from tumour invasion of venous system), **infected vegetations** (from tricuspid endocarditis) and **foreign materials** (from contamination of drugs injected by drug misusers).

Pulmonary hypertension

In normal lungs the pulmonary arterial pressure is about 20/8 mmHg (compared with typical systemic artery systolic/diastolic pressures of 120/80 mmHg) and the mean pulmonary artery pressure is 12–15 mmHg. Pulmonary hypertension is defined as a mean pulmonary artery pressure >25 mmHg at rest. It may occur as a result of hypoxaemia and chronic lung disease, when it is often referred to as **cor pulmonale**, but in some cases there is no demonstrable cause and this is termed **idiopathic pulmonary hypertension**.

Cor pulmonale

Some confusion arises from the differing ways in which this term is used but it essentially refers to the development of pulmonary hypertension and right ventricular hypertrophy secondary to disease of the lungs. **Hypoxaemia** is a powerful stimulus for pulmonary vasoconstriction and this is the most common mechanism giving rise to cor pulmonale (e.g. chronic hypercapnic respiratory failure in COPD). Other mechanisms giving rise to pulmonary hypertension include **vascular obstruction** (e.g. chronic pulmonary emboli, pulmonary artery stenosis), **increased blood flow** (e.g. left-to-right intracardiac shunts—atrial and ventricular septal defects) and **loss of pulmonary vascular bed** (e.g. fibrotic lung disease, emphysema).

The clinical features of cor pulmonale are **elevation of jugular venous pressure**, **hepatomegaly** (as a result of congestion), peripheral **oedema**, a prominent left **parasternal heave**, a **loud pulmonary secondary sound** and a systolic murmur of **tricuspid regurgitation**. A chest X-ray may show large pulmonary arteries with pruning of the vessels in the lung fields. ECG typically shows p pulmonale (tall p wave in leads II III AVF) with a tall R wave in V_1 and ST segment depression with T-wave inversion in $V_1–V_3$. Echocardiography can assess the structure and dimension of the right heart chambers and the pulmonary artery pressure can be estimated from the velocity of the tricuspid regurgitation jet.

Idiopathic pulmonary hypertension

This is a rare disease, affecting about two per million of the population per annum, in which pulmonary hypertension occurs **without a demonstrable cause**. It particularly affects young women. Some cases of familial pulmonary hypertension are inherited as an autosomal dominant trait due to mutations in the bone morphogenetic protein receptor 2 gene. Some cases are associated with human immunodeficiency virus (**HIV**) infection or with use of **appetite-suppressant drugs** (e.g. aminorex, fenfluramine) but in most cases no cause is apparent. Pulmonary hypertension also occurs as a complication of **collagen vascular diseases** such as systemic sclerosis (scleroderma), mixed connective tissue disease and systemic lupus erythematosus (SLE). Some patients with generalised systemic sclerosis develop severe pulmonary fibrosis (see Chapter 14) but there is also a limited cutaneous variant of systemic sclerosis characterised by subcutaneous calcinosis, Raynaud's phenomenon, oesophageal involvement, and sclerodactyly and telangiectasia (CREST syndrome). Patients with the CREST syndrome usually have anti-centromere antibodies and may develop pulmonary hypertension as a primary vascular phenomenon, often in the absence of significant pulmonary fibrosis. Patients present with dyspnoea, fatigue, angina and syncope on exertion. Investigations (e.g. echocardiography, V/Q scans, pulmonary artery catheterisation) are particularly directed towards excluding other causes of pulmonary hypertension such as left-to-right cardiac shunts and chronic thromboembolic disease. The pathophysiology of the disease involves pulmonary artery vasoconstriction, vascular wall remodelling and thrombosis in situ. Treatment of patients with pulmonary hypertension is complex and is delivered from specialist centres. Supportive treatments include warfarin, diuretics, digoxin and oxygen therapy. Pulmonary endarterectomy may be appropriate for some patients with chronic thromboembolic disease. Calcium channel blocker drugs (e.g. nifedipine) produce useful vasodilatation in a small number of these patients. Prostacycline drugs produce vascular smooth muscle relaxation and inhibit vascular smooth muscle growth, and include epoprostenol given as a continuous intravenous infusion via an indwelling central venous catheter, iloprost which is given by inhalation and treprostinil given as a subcutaneous infusion. Endothelial receptor antagonists (e.g. bosentan) reduce vascular tone and proliferation in pulmonary hypertension. Selective phosphodiesterase-5-inhibitors (e.g. sildenafil) also reduce pulmonary artery pressure. Atrial septostomy involves the creation of a right-to-left interatrial shunt and can be used to decompress the failing right heart. Heart–lung or lung transplantation also needs to be considered as the disease is usually progressive.

Pulmonary vasculitis

When pulmonary vasculitis occurs it is usually as part of a more widespread systemic vasculitis such as Wegener's granulomatosis, polyarteritis nodosa, Churg–Strauss syndrome, Goodpasture's disease or collagen vascular diseases (e.g. scleroderma, SLE; see also Chapter 14).

Wegener's granulomatosis

This is characterised by necrotising granulomatous inflammation and vasculitis affecting in particular the **upper airways** (rhinitis, sinusitis, bloodstained nasal discharge), the **lungs** (cavitating nodules, endobronchial disease) and **kidneys** (glomerulonephritis). **Anti-neutrophil cytoplasmic antibodies** (ANCA) are usually present in the serum. It is treated with a combination of corticosteroids and cyclophosphamide.

Churg–Strauss syndrome

This is an unusual disease consisting of allergic granulomatosis and angiitis. It consists of an initial phase of **asthma** followed by marked peripheral blood **eosinophilia** and **eosinophilic vasculitis** giving rise to pulmonary infiltrates, myocarditis, myositis, neuritis, rashes and glomerulonephritis. It usually responds rapidly to corticosteroids.

Polyarteritis nodosa

This consists of a vasculitis of medium and small arteries resulting in **aneurysm** formation, **glomerulonephritis** and **vasculitic lesions** in various organs. Pulmonary involvement is unusual but may result in haemoptysis, pulmonary haemorrhage, fibrosis and pleurisy. There is often considerable overlap in the clinical features of the various vasculitic syndromes.

Goodpasture's syndrome

This consists of a combination of **glomerulonephritis** and **alveolar haemorrhage** in association with circulating **anti-basement membrane antibody** which binds to lung and renal tissue. Pulmonary involvement is more common in smokers and may cause severe pulmonary haemorrhage resulting in haemoptysis, infiltrates on chest X-ray, hypoxaemia and anaemia. Transfer factor may be elevated because of binding of the inhaled carbon monoxide to haemoglobin in the alveoli. Treatment consists of corticosteroids and cyclophosphamide, with plasmapheresis to remove circulating antibodies.

Keypoints

- Most pulmonary emboli arise from thrombosis in the deep veins of the legs, which is common in immobilised patients in the community and in hospital on medical, surgical and obstetric wards.
- Assessing patients with suspected pulmonary emboli involves an appraisal of compatible clinical features and risk factors, exclusion of alternative diagnoses and measurement of D-dimer levels.
- CTPA is increasingly being used as the main imaging modality to confirm or exclude the diagnosis of pulmonary embolism.
- Heparin is used to achieve rapid anti-coagulation, followed by warfarin. Thrombolytic therapy is only given to patients with circulatory compromise from a massive pulmonary embolism.
- Pulmonary hypertension (mean pressure >25 mmHg) may arise from chronic thromboembolic disease, as a result of chronic hypoxic lung disease, or in the form of idiopathic pulmonary hypertension.

Further reading

Blann AD, Lip GYH. Venous thromboembolism. *BMJ* 2006; **332**: 215–19.

British Thoracic Society guidelines for the management of suspected acute pulmonary embolism. *Thorax* 2003; **58**: 470–84.

Ghuysen A, Ghaye B, Willems V. Computed tomographic pulmonary angiography and prognostic significance in patients with acute pulmonary embolism. *Thorax* 2005; **60**: 956–61.

Pulmonary hypertension association. www. pha-uk.com

Robinson GV. Pulmonary embolism in hospital practice. *BMJ* 2006; **332**: 156–60.

Rubin LJ. Pulmonary arterial hypertension. *Proc Am Thorac Soc* 2006; **3**: 111–15.

Chapter 17

Pneumothorax and pleural effusion

Pneumothorax

Pneumothorax is the presence of air in the pleural space. Usually the air enters the pleural space as the result of a leak from a hole in the underlying lung, but rarely it enters from outside as a result of a penetrating chest injury. Pneumothoraces may be classified as **spontaneous** or **traumatic**, and spontaneous pneumothoraces may be **primary**, without evidence of other lung disease, or occur **secondary** to underlying lung disease (e.g. chronic obstructive pulmonary disease (COPD), cystic fibrosis).

Pathogenesis

Spontaneous primary pneumothorax typically occurs in a previously healthy young adult and is most common in tall thin men. Most seem to arise from the rupture of **subpleural blebs or bullae** at the apex of an otherwise normal lung. The aetiology of these blebs is uncertain but they may represent congenital lesions aggravated by the more negative pleural space pressure at the apex of the lung. Smoking is associated with a greatly increased risk of pneumothorax. The intrapleural pressure is normally negative because of the retractive force of lung elastic recoil so that when a communication is established between the atmosphere and the pleural space air is sucked in and the lung deflates. A small hole in the lung often closes off as the lung

deflates. Sometimes the hole remains open and the air leak will then continue until the pressure equalises. Occasionally, the opening from the lung to the pleural space functions as a valve allowing air to leak into the pleural space during inspiration but not to re-enter the lung on expiration. This is a potentially lethal situation as the air accumulates in the pleural space under increasing pressure giving a **tension pneumothorax** in which the lung is pushed down, the mediastinum is shifted to the opposite side and the venous return to the heart and cardiac output are impaired.

There is an increased risk of pneumothorax in association with virtually all lung diseases. These spontaneous secondary pneumothoraces are particularly common in patients with COPD and bullous emphysema. A pneumothorax resulting from rupture of a bulla may render an already disabled patient critically ill. Pneumothorax is a well-recognised complication of positive pressure endotracheal ventilation on intensive therapy units (ITUs) of patients with underlying lung disease. Traumatic pneumothorax usually arises from puncture of the lung by a fractured rib but air may enter the pleural space from outside via a penetrating injury or from rupture of alveoli, oesophagus, trachea or bronchi. **Iatrogenic** ('doctor-induced') pneumothorax may arise as a complication of invasive chest procedures such as the insertion of a catheter into the subclavian vein, percutaneous needle aspiration of a lung lesion or transbronchial lung biopsy.

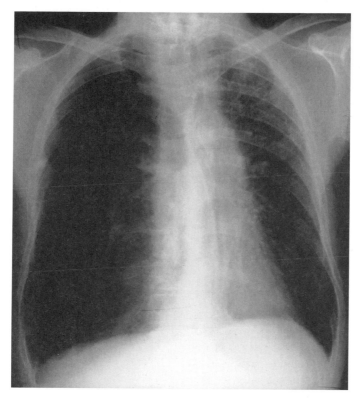

Figure 17.1 This 55-year-old man with chronic perihilar fibrosis caused by sarcoidosis developed acute dyspnoea and right pleuritic pain followed by increasing respiratory distress. On arrival in hospital examination showed diminished breath sounds and hyper-resonance over the right lung, with deviation of the trachea to the left. Chest X-ray shows a right tension pneumothorax with a large gas-filled pleural space without lung markings in the right hemithorax, deflation of the right lung and shift of the mediastinum to the left. He was given oxygen and analgesia, and an intercostal chest tube was inserted into the right pleural space as an emergency procedure, with successful re-expansion of the lung and relief of his respiratory distress.

Clinical features

Pneumothorax typically presents with acute **pleuritic pain** and **breathlessness**. An otherwise healthy young adult may tolerate a pneumothorax quite well but older patients with underlying lung disease often develop severe respiratory distress with cyanosis. The clinical signs of pneumothorax are **reduced breath sounds** and **hyper-resonance** on the side of the pneumothorax, but these may be difficult to detect. Sometimes a left-sided pneumothorax is associated with a clicking noise if the cardiac beat produces friction on movement of the layers of the pleura. Signs of **mediastinal shift** such as displacement of the trachea and apex beat to the

opposite side may be detectable in a tension pneumothorax.

The **chest X-ray** shows a black gas space, containing no lung markings, between the margin of the collapsed lung and the chest wall (Fig. 17.1). Typically the visceral pleura of the margin of the lung is visible as a laterally convex 'pleural line' which runs parallel to the chest wall and the pulmonary vascular markings are absent lateral to this line. Identification of a convex pleural line helps to differentiate a pneumothorax from a large bulla (see Chapter 12, Fig. 12.5). A chest X-ray taken after expiration may accentuate the radiological features and may help to detect a small pneumothorax but expiratory X-rays are not

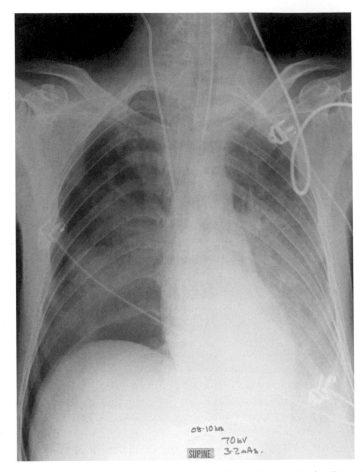

Figure 17.2 Chest X-ray of a pneumothorax in a patient lying flat. This patient was in the ITU receiving endotracheal ventilation. His condition deteriorated with hypoxia, tachycardia and hypotension. The chest X-ray shows an endotracheal tube in satisfactory position, a cannula in the right internal jugular vein, left lower lobe consolidation and evidence of a right pneumothorax. When a patient with a pneumothorax is lying flat the air in the pleural space tends to collect anteriorly and inferiorly giving the appearance of hyperlucency with unusual clarity of the mediastinal contour and the costophrenic angle, and the typical 'pleural line' at the margin of the lung, which is characteristic of a pneumothorax in an upright patient, is often not present.

needed routinely. It is often difficult to detect a pneumothorax if the chest X-ray is performed with the patient lying supine (e.g. on ventilation in the ITU) because the air in the pleural space, in this position, rises anteriorly giving an appearance of hyperlucency of the lower chest, such that the mediastinal contours and costophrenic angle are outlined with increased clarity (Fig. 17.2). If the patient cannot be imaged in an upright position, a lateral decubitus film should be performed. The size of a pneumothorax can be quantified arbitrarily as being 'small' if the rim of air between the margin of the collapsed lung and chest wall is, <2 cm, or 'large' if it is ⩾2 cm. The volume of a 2 cm rim of air is approximately a 50% pneumothorax.

Treatment

● *No intervention*: A small (rim of air <2 cm) pneumothorax which is not causing respiratory distress may not require any intervention because it will **resolve spontaneously at a rate of about**

1–2% per day. Such patients may be allowed home with advice to return to hospital immediately if symptoms deteriorate. They should not undertake an airplane flight until 1 week after the chest X-ray shows complete resolution of the pneumothorax because the reduced barometric pressure at altitude causes expansion of enclosed thoracic air pockets. A follow-up appointment should be arranged for clinical assessment and chest X-ray to ensure resolution of the pneumothorax and to exclude underlying lung disease. If a patient with a pneumothorax is admitted to hospital for observation **high-flow oxygen** (e.g. 10 L/min) should be administered, with appropriate caution in patients with COPD who may be sensitive to higher concentrations of oxygen. Inhalation of oxygen reduces the total pressure of gases in the pleural capillaries by reducing the partial pressure of nitrogen. This increases the pressure gradient between the pleural capillaries and the pleural cavity and increases absorption of air from the pneumothorax.

• *Aspiration*: Air may be aspirated from the pleural space by inserting a French gauge 16 cannula (such as an intravenous cannula) through the second intercostal space in the mid-clavicular line after injection of local anaesthetic. Once the pleural cavity is entered, the needle is removed and the cannula is connected via a three-way tip to a syringe, and air is aspirated. A chest X-ray is performed to assess the success of the procedure. This technique is simple, less distressing to the patient than insertion of a chest tube, and very effective for primary pneumothoraces. Even large pneumothoraces can be aspirated but it is less successful for secondary pneumothoraces and chest tube insertion is needed if aspiration is unsuccessful, if there is a persistent air leak from the lung or if there is a tension pneumothorax.

• *Intercostal tube drainage* (Fig. 17.3): Intercostal tube drainage is needed for most secondary pneumothoraces (i.e. in patients with underlying lung disease e.g. COPD) or where simple aspiration has failed.

Small calibre (e.g. size 12–20 F) tubes (Fig. 17.3a) can be passed into the pleural space to drain air or fluid using a **Seldinger technique** whereby, after injection of local anaesthetic, a guide wire is inserted via a specially designed cannula and then the tube is passed over the guide-wire into the pleural space. The tube is sutured in place and attached to an underwater seal. These small calibre tubes are very effective at draining air and fluid from the pleural space and they cause less pain and discomfort to the patient than the conventional large calibre tubes.

Large calibre (e.g. size 24–32 F) tubes (Fig. 17.3b) are needed if there is a very large air leak from the lung which exceeds the capacity of the smaller tubes. The insertion of a chest tube is a frightening procedure for the patient, who needs adequate **explanation and reassurance**. Pre-medication with atropine (300–600 µg intravenously) prevents vasovagal reactions, and a small dose of a sedative (e.g. midazolam 1–2 mg intravenously) may be considered for very anxious patients. The chest X-ray should be studied to confirm the correct side and location for insertion of the tube. This is usually the fourth, fifth or sixth intercostal space in the mid-axillary line. Sterile gloves are worn and the skin is cleaned with antiseptic solution. The skin, subcutaneous tissues, intercostal muscles and parietal pleura are anaesthetised by injection of 10–20 ml of 1% **lidocaine (lignocaine)**. Aspiration of air into the syringe confirms that the pleural space has been entered. The skin is incised and **blunt dissection** with a forceps is used to make a track through the intercostal muscles into the pleural space, taking care to avoid the neurovascular bundle situated in the groove on the lower surface of each rib. The chest tube may then be inserted through the track, guided by a forceps or by a trocar which can be helpful in directing the tube towards the apex. The track made by blunt dissection should be sufficiently wide to **allow the drain to slide in easily without force**, and care must be taken to avoid causing damage to the underlying lung or other structures. The tube is securely **anchored in place** with a suture and connected to an underwater seal. The end of the tube should be 2–3 cm below the level of the water in the bottle. **Oscillation** of the meniscus of the water in the tube indicates that the tube is patent and in the pleural space. **Bubbling** on respiration or coughing indicates

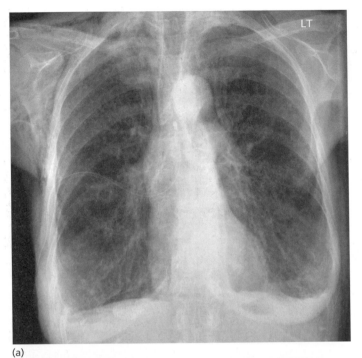

(a)

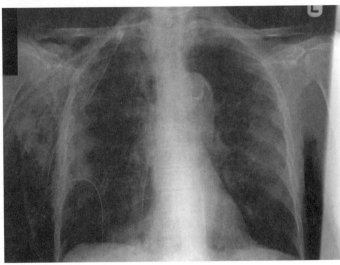

(b)

Figure 17.3 (a) Chest X-ray showing a small calibre tube which was inserted using a Seldinger technique (tube passed over a guide-wire) into the pleural space of a patient who had suffered a right spontaneous primary pneumothorax which had failed to resolve on simple aspiration. (b) Chest X-ray showing two large calibre tubes which were inserted by blunt dissection, in a patient with COPD who had suffered a secondary pneumothorax with a large air leak. Air has tracked into the tissues of the right chest wall causing 'subcutaneous emphysema'.

continued drainage of air. Breathing with a chest tube in place is painful and **adequate analgesia** should be prescribed. The position of the tube and the degree of re-expansion of the lung should be checked by chest X-ray.

Low-pressure (-10 to $-20\,\text{cmH}_2\text{O}$) suction applied to the tube may expedite the removal of air.

• *Surgical intervention*: Surgical treatment is required for persistent or recurrent pneumothoraces. Failure of re-expansion of the lung with profuse bubbling of air through the underwater drain suggests a bronchopleural fistula (i.e. a persistent communication between the lung and pleural space). **Surgical closure of the hole** with pleurodesis is

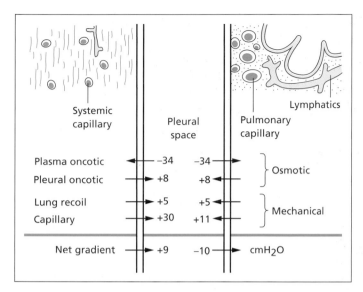

Figure 17.4 Pleural fluid dynamics. In the normal pleural space the mechanical and oncotic pressures are in equilibrium such that net filtration of fluid by the parietal pleura is balanced by net absorption of fluid by the visceral pleura. Pleural effusion may arise from changes in the mechanical and oncotic pressures (transudates) or from increased capillary permeability brought about by disease of the pleura (exudates).

usually necessary and may be performed via a thoracotomy or via thoracoscopy. The hole is oversewn and blebs on the surface of the lung are excised. **Pleurodesis** involves the obliteration of the pleural space and can be achieved by instilling tetracycline or talc which provokes adhesions between the visceral and parietal pleura. **Pleurectomy** involves the removal of the parietal pleura. Usually, an apicolateral pleurectomy (leaving the posterobasal pleura intact) prevents recurrence without compromising lung function. There is quite a high risk of recurrence after a first spontaneous primary pneumothorax, with about 50% of patients suffering a second pneumothorax within 4 years. Surgical intervention is usually recommended after a second pneumothorax. This is also the case if the patient has suffered a pneumothorax on both sides, because of the risk of catastrophic simultaneous bilateral pneumothoraces. Particular thought must be given to the best procedure for young adults with complicated pneumothoraces secondary to diseases such as cystic fibrosis so as not to compromise potential future lung transplantation. A limited apicolateral surgical abrasion pleurodesis may be the best option in these circumstances.

Pleural effusion

A pleural effusion is a collection of fluid in the pleural space.

Pleural fluid dynamics

The parietal and visceral pleural surfaces are normally in close contact and the potential space between them contains only a very thin layer of fluid. Pleural fluid dynamics are complex and incompletely understood but Fig. 17.4 shows, in a simplified form, some of the main factors governing fluid filtration and absorption. The parietal pleura is perfused by the systemic circulation, and the high systemic capillary pressure, negative intrapleural pressure and pleural oncotic pressure overcome the plasma oncotic pressure resulting in fluid filtration into the pleural space. The visceral pleura is mainly perfused by the pulmonary circulation with its low pulmonary capillary pressure so that the balance of forces results in movement of fluid outward from the pleural space to the veins and lymphatics. The balance between **fluid filtration** by the parietal pleura and **fluid absorption** by the visceral pleura is

185

such that fluid does not normally collect in the pleural space. Pleural effusions may develop from **increased capillary pressure** (e.g. left ventricular failure), **reduced plasma oncotic pressure** (e.g. hypoalbuminaemia), **increased capillary permeability** (e.g. disease of pleura) or **obstruction of lymphatic drainage** (e.g. carcinoma of lymphatics).

Clinical features

Patients with pleural effusions typically present with **dyspnoea**, sometimes with pleuritic pain, and often with features of associated diseases (e.g. cardiac failure, carcinoma, etc.). The signs of pleural effusion are **decreased expansion** on the side of the effusion, **stony dullness, diminished breath sounds** and **reduced tactile vocal fremitus**. Sometimes **bronchial breathing** is heard at the upper level of the fluid. In taking the patient's history it is important to enquire about clues to possible causes of pleural effusion such as asbestos exposure, contact with tuberculosis, smoking, drugs (e.g. dantrolene, bromocriptine) or systemic disease. A full careful physical examination is essential to detect signs of underlying disease (e.g. cardiac failure, breast lump, lymphadenopathy, etc.).

Investigations (Fig. 17.5)

- *Radiology*: **Chest X-ray** characteristically shows a dense white shadow with a concave upper edge (Fig. 17.6). Small effusions cause no more than blunting of a costophrenic angle whereas very large effusions cause 'white out' of an entire hemithorax with shift of the mediastinum to the opposite side. Pleural fluid can be difficult to detect if the chest X-ray is performed with the patient lying supine, and may only be suspected by haziness on the affected side. A **lateral decubitus** film may be useful in demonstrating mobility of the fluid, distinguishing the features from pleural thickening. **Ultrasound** imaging is helpful in localising loculated effusions and in positioning chest tubes. **Computed tomography (CT)** may be helpful in detecting pleural tumours (e.g. mesothelioma) and in assessing the underlying lung and mediastinum.

- *Pleural fluid aspiration (thoracocentesis)* is the key initial investigation. A **protein** level >30 g/L and **lactate dehydrogenase (LDH)** level >200 iu/L indicate that the effusion is an exudate and that further investigations for pleural disease are indicated. Both transudates and exudates are typically a yellow, straw colour. **Bloodstained** fluid points towards malignancy, pulmonary infarction or severe inflammation. **Pus** indicates an empyema, **milky** white fluid suggests a chylothorax and frank **blood** suggests a haemothorax (e.g. as a result of trauma). A low **glucose** content points towards infection or a connective tissue disease as a cause of the effusion. A high **amylase** content is characteristic of pleural effusion associated with pancreatitis but also sometimes occurs with adenocarcinoma. **Neutrophils** are the predominant cells in acute inflammation or infection and **lymphocytes** in chronic effusions particularly caused by tuberculosis or malignancy. **Cytology** may show malignant cells (e.g. mesothelioma or metastatic carcinoma).

  Microbiology examination of the fluid may identify tuberculosis or bacterial infection, for example.

- *Pleural biopsy* may be performed using a specially designed needle such as the **Abram's needle**. After injection of local anaesthetic, incision of the skin and blunt dissection of the intercostal muscles, the needle is passed into the pleural space. The Abram's needle is in two parts which can be rotated on each other; pleural fluid can be aspirated when the window of the needle is rotated to the open position. The needle is then pulled back until some parietal pleural tissue is caught in the notch of the needle. The inner cylinder of the needle has a sharp cutting edge which when rotated cuts off pleural tissue caught in the notch (Fig. 17.5). **Radiologically guided biopsy** is particularly useful in diagnosing malignant disease of the pleura when CT has shown a focal area of pleural thickening. Histology of pleural biopsy samples is particularly useful in diagnosing malignant effusions or tuberculosis (e.g. caseating granuloma). A sample of the biopsy should also be sent for culture for *Mycobacterium tuberculosis*. **Video-assisted thoracoscopy**, which is usually performed under general anaesthesia,

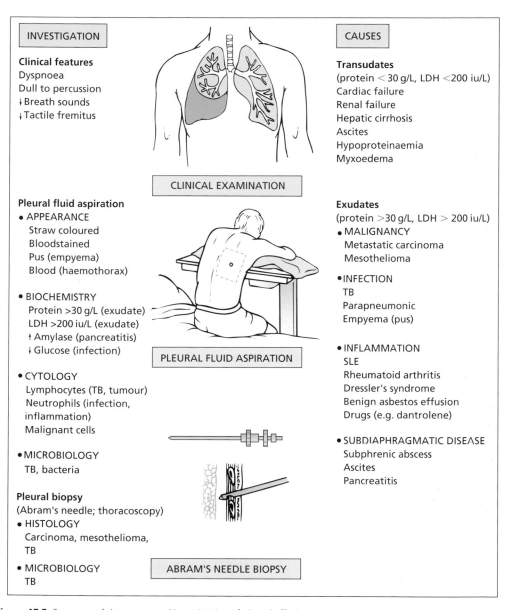

INVESTIGATION

Clinical features
Dyspnoea
Dull to percussion
↓Breath sounds
↓Tactile fremitus

CLINICAL EXAMINATION

Pleural fluid aspiration
- APPEARANCE
  Straw coloured
  Bloodstained
  Pus (empyema)
  Blood (haemothorax)

- BIOCHEMISTRY
  Protein >30 g/L (exudate)
  LDH >200 iu/L (exudate)
  ↑ Amylase (pancreatitis)
  ↓ Glucose (infection)

- CYTOLOGY
  Lymphocytes (TB, tumour)
  Neutrophils (infection, inflammation)
  Malignant cells

- MICROBIOLOGY
  TB, bacteria

Pleural biopsy
(Abram's needle; thoracoscopy)
- HISTOLOGY
  Carcinoma, mesothelioma, TB

- MICROBIOLOGY
  TB

PLEURAL FLUID ASPIRATION

ABRAM'S NEEDLE BIOPSY

CAUSES

Transudates
(protein < 30 g/L, LDH <200 iu/L)
Cardiac failure
Renal failure
Hepatic cirrhosis
Ascites
Hypoproteinaemia
Myxoedema

Exudates
(protein >30 g/L, LDH > 200 iu/L)
- MALIGNANCY
  Metastatic carcinoma
  Mesothelioma

- INFECTION
  TB
  Parapneumonic
  Empyema (pus)

- INFLAMMATION
  SLE
  Rheumatoid arthritis
  Dressler's syndrome
  Benign asbestos effusion
  Drugs (e.g. dantrolene)

- SUBDIAPHRAGMATIC DISEASE
  Subphrenic abscess
  Ascites
  Pancreatitis

Figure 17.5 Summary of the causes and investigation of pleural effusions.

allows direct inspection of the pleural surfaces with direct biopsy of abnormal tissue.

Further investigations (e.g. bronchoscopy for suspected lung carcinoma or ultrasound of abdomen for suspected subphrenic disease) may be required depending on the clues to diagnosis elicited on initial assessment.

Causes

Pleural effusions are classified as transudates or exudates. Transudates are characterised by a low protein content (<30 g/L) and a low LDH level (<200 iu/L). They arise as a result of changes in hydrostatic or osmotic pressures across the pleural

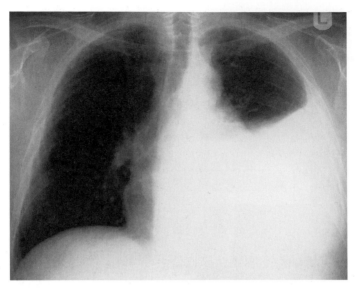

Figure 17.6 This 68-year-old man presented with a 6-week history of progressive breathlessness and left pleuritic pain. On examination there was stony dullness and diminished breath sounds over the left hemithorax. The chest X-ray shows features of a large pleural effusion with a dense white shadow with a concave upper border over the left side of the chest. The pleural fluid was bloodstained and showed metastatic adenocarcinoma on cytology. Bronchoscopy showed the primary tumour partly occluding the left lower lobe bronchus. An intercostal drain was inserted to evacuate the fluid and tetracycline was instilled to achieve pleurodesis.

membrane rather than from disease of the pleura. Exudates are characterised by a high protein (>30 g/L) and LDH (>200 iu/L) content, and result from increased permeability associated with disease of the pleura. Sometimes, in patients with borderline protein and LDH levels, there is difficulty in distinguishing between transudates and exudates, and comparison of pleural to serum ratios may be helpful: exudates have a pleural fluid/serum protein ratio >0.5 and an LDH ratio >0.6.

Transudates

The main causes of transudative pleural effusions are **cardiac failure**, **renal failure**, **hepatic cirrhosis** and **hypoproteinaemia** caused by malnutrition or nephrotic syndrome, for example. In most cases transudative effusions are bilateral, although they may be asymmetrical and initially unilateral. **Ascitic fluid** may pass through pleuroperitoneal communications, which are more common in the right hemidiaphragm. Similarly, **peritoneal dialysis fluid** may give rise to a right pleural effusion.

Rare causes of transudates are **myxoedema** and Meigs' syndrome (benign ovarian fibroma, ascites and pleural effusion, which may be a transudate or exudate). Sometimes, treatment of cardiac failure with diuretics results in an increase in fluid protein content so that the effusion appears to be an exudate. Treatment of transudates involves correction of the underlying hydrostatic or osmotic mechanisms (e.g. treatment of cardiac failure or hypoproteinaemia), and further investigation of the pleura is not usually necessary.

Exudates

A variety of diseases that affect the pleura are associated with increased capillary permeability or reduced lymphatic drainage. Exudates are often unilateral and investigations are directed towards identifying the cause because this determines treatment.
• *Malignancy*: **Metastases** to the pleura most commonly arise from **lung**, **breast**, **ovarian** or **gastrointestinal** cancers and from **lymphoma**.

Mesothelioma is a primary tumour of the pleura related to asbestos exposure (see Chapter 15). In malignant effusions the fluid is often bloodstained with a high lymphocyte count, and cytology often shows malignant cells. If cytology of a pleural aspirate is negative, pleural biopsy may be diagnostic. Sometimes, confirmation of the diagnosis is difficult and thoracoscopy with biopsy of lesions under direct vision may be necessary. Malignancy may give rise to pleural effusions by means other than direct involvement of the pleura. **Lymphatic involvement** by tumours may obstruct drainage and cause pleural effusions with negative cytology. **Chylous effusions**, caused by malignancy in the thoracic duct, are characterised by a milky cloudy appearance of the pleural fluid. **Superior vena caval obstruction** may give rise to pleural effusions as a result of elevation of systemic venous pressure. Treatment of a pleural effusion associated with malignancy is directed against the underlying tumour (e.g. chemotherapy). **Drainage of the fluid** by needle aspiration or intercostal chest tube relieves dyspnoea. It is usually advisable to remove the fluid slowly at no more than 1–1.5 L at a time as too rapid removal may provoke re-expansion pulmonary oedema, although the risk is small. The risk of recurrence of the effusion may be reduced by the instillation of a sclerosing agent (e.g. tetracycline 1–1.5 g, doxycycline 500 mg or sterile talc 2–5 g in 50 mL saline) into the pleural space to provoke chemical **pleurodesis**. Lidocaine (lignocaine) 3 mg/kg, maximum 250 mg may be instilled intrapleurally before the sclerosing agent to provide local anaesthesia. It is important that the effusion has been drained to dryness before insertion of the sclerosing agent so that the two pleural surfaces can be apposed so as to promote adhesions. If chemical pleurodesis is not successful, surgical pleurodesis or **pleurectomy via thoracoscopy** may be helpful.

• *Infection*: Pneumonia may be complicated by an inflammatory reaction in the pleura resulting in a **parapneumonic effusion**. Secondary infection of this effusion with multiplication of bacteria in the pleural space produces an **empyema** which is the presence of pus in the pleural cavity. If a parapneumonic effusion has a low pH (<7.2) there is a high risk of an empyema developing and early tube drainage is indicated. Various organisms may give rise to an empyema including *Streptococcus pneumoniae*, *Staphylococcus aureus*, *Streptococcus milleri* and anaerobic organisms (e.g. *Bacteroides*). Empyema is particularly associated with aspiration pneumonia (e.g. related to unconsciousness, alcohol, vomiting, dysphagia, etc.). **Actinomycosis** is an unusual infection which spreads from the lung to the pleura and chest wall with a tendency to form sinus tracts. **Tuberculosis** must always be borne in mind as a cause of pleural effusion or empyema (see Chapter 7).

Initial **antibiotic treatment** is often with amoxicillin and metronidazole, adjusted in accordance with results of microbiology tests. The key treatment of empyema, however, is **drainage of the pus**. Placement of the drainage tube is often best guided by ultrasound imaging as the effusion is often loculated as a result of fibrin deposition and adhesions. Instillation of a **fibrinolytic agent** (e.g. streptokinase 250 000 units or urokinase 100 000 units in 20 mL of saline, left in situ for 2 hours, daily for 3–5 days) through the chest tube into the pleural space is sometimes used to improve drainage by promoting lysis of fibrin adhesions. It may be effective in selected patients with empyema but it is not recommended routinely for all patients. **Surgical intervention** is necessary if these measures fail and a variety of approaches may be used including rib resection with open drainage, or thoracotomy with removal of infected debris and decortication (stripping of the pleura and empyematous sac).

• *Inflammatory diseases*: Various inflammatory diseases may involve the pleura. Effusions associated with **connective tissue diseases** (e.g. rheumatoid arthritis, systemic lupus erythematosus) characteristically have a low glucose content. **Drug reactions** involving the pleura have been described with dantrolene, bromocriptine, nitrofurantoin and methysergide, for example. **Asbestos** may give rise to **benign asbestos-related pleural effusions** which may recur producing diffuse pleural thickening (see Chapter 15). Small pleural effusions may complicate **pulmonary embolism** and infarction (see Chapter 16). **Dressler's syndrome** consists of inflammatory pericarditis and pleurisy of uncertain aetiology following a myocardial infarction or cardiac surgery.

- *Subdiaphragmatic disease*: **Pancreatitis** may be associated with pleural effusions probably as a result of diaphragmatic inflammation. Such effusions are usually left sided and characterised by a high amylase content. **Ascites** may traverse the diaphragm through pleuroperitoneal communications causing a pleural effusion. Spread of infection or inflammation from a **subphrenic abscess** or **intrahepatic abscess** may also cause a pleural effusion.

Oesophageal rupture

Oesophageal rupture may give rise to a pyopneumothorax (air and pus in the pleural cavity). This may result from external **trauma** or be **iatrogenic** (e.g. perforation during endoscopy). **Spontaneous rupture of the oesophagus** (Boerhaave's syndrome) is a rare but catastrophic condition which typically occurs when the patient attempts to suppress vomiting by closure of the pharyngeal sphincter. Intraoesophageal pressure rises steeply and rupture typically occurs in the lowest third of the oesophagus. It is a more severe form of the Mallory–Weiss syndrome of haematemesis caused by mucosal tears from protracted vomiting. Characteristically, vomiting is followed by chest pain and subcutaneous emphysema (palpable air in skin) as air and gastric contents leak into the mediastinum. A few hours later the pleural membrane gives way and air and food debris pass into the pleural cavity producing pleuritic pain, pleural effusion and empyema. Chest X-ray typically shows an initial pneumomediastinum (a rim of air around mediastinal structures) followed by a hydropneumothorax. The diagnosis is notoriously difficult to make and a radiocontrast oesophagogram is the key investigation. Thoracotomy with repair of the oesophagus is usually the best treatment.

Keypoints

- Pneumothorax is the presence of air in the pleural space and this usually occurs from rupture of subpleural cysts in the underlying lung.
- A small pneumothorax (<2 cm rim of air) may not require intervention. A larger pneumothorax (>2 cm rim of air) is treated by simple aspiration or insertion of an intercostal tube.
- A pleural effusion is a collection of fluid in the pleural space.
- Transudative effusions result from changes in hydrostatic pressure (e.g. cardiac failure). Exudative effusions result from diseases of the pleura (e.g. malignancy, infection, inflammation).
- Investigation of an exudative effusion involves clinical assessment, imaging (e.g. CT), pleural fluid aspiration (for biochemistry, cytology and microbiology) and pleural biopsy.

Further reading

Bouros D, Antoniou KM, Light RW. Intrapleural streptokinase for pleural infection. *BMJ* 2006; **332**: 133–4.

British Thoracic Society guidelines for the management of pleural disease. *Thorax* 2003; **58** (Suppl II): 1–59.

Henry MT. Simple sequential treatment for primary spontaneous pneumothorax: one step closer. *Eur Resp J* 2006; **27**: 448–50.

Light RW. Parapneumonic effusions and empyema. *Proc Am Thorac Soc* 2005; **3**: 75–80.

Tokuda y, Matsushima D, Stein GH, Miyagi S. Intrapleural fibrinolytic agents for empyema and complicated parapneumonic effusions. *Chest* 2006; **129**: 783–90.

Chapter 18

Acute respiratory distress syndrome

Introduction

The acute respiratory distress syndrome (ARDS) is a form of **acute respiratory failure** caused by **permeability pulmonary oedema** resulting from **endothelial damage** due to a cascade of **inflammatory events** developing in response to an **initiating injury or illness**.

It had long been recognised that soldiers wounded in battle often died of respiratory failure some days later. During World Wars I and II it was thought that this was because of lung infection or excessive fluid administration. Further experience of the condition during the Vietnam War showed that despite successful surgical management of wounds and optimal fluid replacement, soldiers were still dying of pulmonary dysfunction some days later and that the lungs showed features such as oedema, atelectasis, haemorrhage and hyaline membrane formation. It was not until 1967 that this condition was recognised as a specific clinical entity separate from the precipitating injury, and that it could also arise from civilian injuries and illnesses. The term adult respiratory distress syndrome was sometimes used because of the superficial similarity of the pathology of the disease, showing hyaline membranes, to the infant respiratory distress syndrome (caused by surfactant deficiency in premature babies), although the term acute respiratory distress syndrome is more appropriate.

Pathogenesis

In most situations pulmonary oedema arises as a result of increased pulmonary capillary **pressure** (e.g. left ventricular failure) but in ARDS it arises because of increased alveolar capillary **permeability**.

Pressure pulmonary oedema (Fig. 18.1)

In the normal situation the hydrostatic pressure and the osmotic pressure exerted by the plasma proteins are in a state of equilibrium between the pulmonary capillaries and lung alveoli. An **increase in hydrostatic pressure** is the most common cause of pulmonary oedema and this typically occurs secondary to elevated left atrial pressure from left ventricular failure (e.g. after myocardial infarction) or from mitral valve disease (e.g. mitral stenosis). **Volume overload** may also increase pulmonary capillary pressure and this may arise from excessive intravenous fluid administration or fluid retention (e.g. renal failure). **Reduced osmotic pressure** may contribute to pulmonary oedema and this occurs in hypoproteinaemic states (e.g. severely ill, malnourished patients; nephrotic syndrome with renal protein loss). In the early stages of pulmonary oedema there is an increase in the fluid content of the interstitial space between the capillaries and alveoli but as the condition deteriorates flooding of the alveoli occurs.

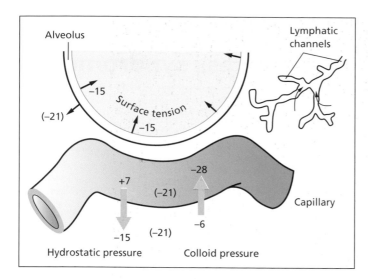

Figure 18.1 Diagram illustrating approximate values for hydrostatic and colloid pressures in millimetres of mercury (mmHg) between the pulmonary capillary and alveolus. Pulmonary oedema may arise from increased **hydrostatic pressure** (e.g. cardiogenic pulmonary oedema), from reduced **colloid pressure** (e.g. hypoalbuminaemia), or from increased capillary **permeability** (e.g. ARDS).

Permeability pulmonary oedema

In ARDS a cascade of inflammatory events arises over a period of hours from a focus of tissue damage. In particular, activated neutrophils aggregate and adhere to endothelial cells, releasing various toxins, oxygen radicals and mediators (e.g. arachidonic acid, histamine, kinins). This **systemic inflammatory response** may be initiated by a variety of injuries or illnesses and gives rise to **acute lung injury** as one of its earliest manifestations, with the development of **endothelial damage** and **increased alveolar capillary permeability**. The alveoli become filled with a protein-rich exudate containing abundant neutrophils and other inflammatory cells and the airspaces show a rim of proteinaceous material—the hyaline membrane. The characteristic feature of permeability pulmonary oedema in ARDS is that the pulmonary capillary wedge pressure is not elevated. This may be measured by passing a special balloon-tipped pulmonary artery catheter (e.g. Swan–Ganz catheter) via a central vein through the right side of the heart to the pulmonary artery. The balloon of the catheter is then inflated and is carried forward in the blood flow until it wedges in a pulmonary capillary. The measurement of pulmonary capillary wedge pressure reflects left atrial pressure and in ARDS it is typically ≤18 mmHg, whereas in cardiogenic pulmonary oedema it is elevated.

Table 18.1 ARDS: initiating injuries and illnesses.

Direct	Indirect
Aspiration of gastric contents	Sepsis
Severe pneumonia	Major trauma
Smoke inhalation	Multiple blood transfusions
Lung contusion	Pancreatitis
Fat embolism	Extensive burns
Amniotic fluid embolism	Anaphylaxis
Chemical inhalation (e.g. silo filler's lung)	Hypotensive shock
Oxygen toxicity/ventilator lung	Disseminated intravascular coagulation

Various illnesses and injuries, which affect the lungs directly or indirectly, initiate a cascade of inflammatory responses resulting in endothelial damage and the characteristic permeability pulmonary oedema of ARDS.

Clinical features

ARDS develops in response to a variety of injuries or illnesses which affect the lungs either **directly** (e.g. aspiration of gastric contents, severe pneumonia, lung contusion) or **indirectly** (e.g. systemic sepsis, major trauma, pancreatitis). About 12–48 hours after an initiating event the patient develops respiratory distress with increasing dyspnoea and tachypnoea. Arterial blood gases show deteriorating

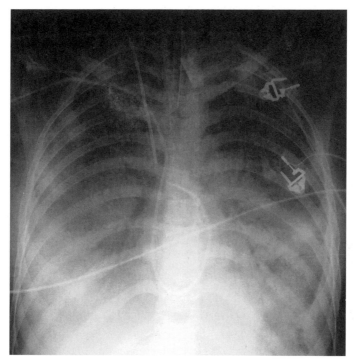

Figure 18.2 This 21-year-old diabetic patient was admitted to the intensive therapy unit (ITU) having vomited and inhaled gastric contents while unconscious with severe ketoacidosis. Despite antibiotics and treatment of ketoacidosis she developed ARDS with progressive respiratory distress and severe hypoxaemia refractory to oxygen therapy. The chest X-ray shows diffuse bilateral shadowing with air bronchograms (black tubes of air against the white background of consolidated lung). An endotracheal tube is in place and the patient is being mechanically ventilated, with a positive end-expiratory pressure (PEEP) of 7.5 cm H_2O. Electrocardiogram monitor leads are visible and a central venous line has been inserted via the right internal jugular vein. A Swan–Ganz catheter has been passed from the right subclavian vein and can be seen, looped around through the right side of the heart into the pulmonary artery. Pulmonary capillary wedge pressure was low at 8 mmHg indicating that the lung shadowing was not caused by cardiogenic pulmonary oedema, but by increased capillary permeability of ARDS. Despite requiring prolonged ventilation and support on ITU the patient made a full recovery.

hypoxaemia which responds poorly to oxygen therapy. Diffuse bilateral infiltrates develop on chest X-ray in the absence of evidence of cardiogenic pulmonary oedema. ARDS is the most severe end of the spectrum of acute lung injury and is characterised by the following features:

- A history of an **initiating injury or illness** (Table 18.1).
- **Hypoxaemia** refractory to oxygen therapy (e.g. $P_{O_2} < 8.0$ kPa (60 mmHg) on 40% oxygen). The degree of hypoxaemia may be expressed as the ratio of arterial oxygen tension (P_{O_2}) to the fractional inspired oxygen concentration ($F_iO_2/100\%$

oxygen = F_iO_2 of 1). In ARDS P_{O_2}/F_iO_2 is < 26 kPa (200 mmHg).

- Bilateral **diffuse infiltrates on chest X-ray** (Fig. 18.2).
- No evidence of cardiogenic pulmonary oedema (e.g. **pulmonary capillary wedge pressure** ≤18 mmHg).

Recognition of critically ill patients

Patients who subsequently develop ARDS may appear deceptively well in the initial stages of their illness. Early recognition and careful observation of

Table 18.2 Features indicating a critically ill patient. A patient demonstrating any of these warning signs needs urgent attention and consideration for ITU care.

Respiratory rate	<8 or >30/min
Pulse rate	<40 or >130/min
Blood pressure	<90 mmHg
Temperature	Hyperthermia (>38°C, 100.4°F)
	Hypothermia (<36°C, 96.8°F)
Urine output	<30 mL/hour for 3 hours
Level of consciousness	Not responding to commands
Oxygenation	O_2 saturation <90% or Pao_2 < 8 kPa (60 mmHg) despite 60% inspired oxygen
Acidosis	pH < 7.2; bicarbonate <20 mmol/L

at-risk patients is of crucial importance in detecting the signs of deterioration and in identifying the need for intensive therapy unit (ITU) care. Certain warning signs are applicable in a wide variety of clinical circumstances because there is often a common physiological pathway of deterioration in the severely ill which can be detected by simple observations of the **pulse rate**, **respiratory rate**, **blood pressure**, **temperature**, **urine output** and **level of consciousness** (Table 18.2). Arterial blood gas measurements provide useful additional information about gas exchange and the metabolic state of the patient.

Treatment

The treatment of ARDS consists of optimal management of the initiating illness or injury combined with supportive care directed at preserving adequate oxygenation, maintaining optimal haemodynamic function and compensating for multiorgan failure which often supervenes.

Treatment of initiating illness

Prompt and complete treatment of the initiating injury or illness is essential. This includes rapid resuscitation with correction of hypotension in patients with multiple trauma for example, and

eradication of any source of sepsis (e.g. intra-abdominal abscess or ischaemic bowel post-surgery).

Respiratory support

Characteristically, the hypoxaemia of ARDS is refractory to **oxygen therapy** because of shunting of blood through areas of lung which are not being ventilated as a result of the alveoli being filled with a proteinaceous exudate and undergoing atelectasis. **Continuous positive airway pressure (CPAP)** can be applied via a tight-fitting nasal mask to prevent alveolar atelectasis and thereby reduce ventilation/perfusion mismatch and the work of breathing. However, **endotracheal intubation and mechanical ventilation** rapidly become necessary and the patient may need to be transferred to a **specialist ITU** with expertise and facilities for treating ARDS. Intermittent positive pressure ventilation mechanically inflates the lungs, delivering oxygen-enriched air at a set tidal volume and rate. Adjustments in the volume, inflation pressure, rate and percentage oxygen are made to achieve adequate ventilation. A **positive end-expiratory pressure (PEEP)** of 5–15 cmH$_2$O is usually applied at the end of the expiratory cycle to prevent collapse of the alveoli. High airway pressures may be generated in ventilating the non-compliant stiff lungs in ARDS and this can reduce cardiac output and carries the risk of barotrauma (e.g. pneumothorax). High ventilation pressures combined with high oxygen concentrations may themselves result in microvascular damage which perpetuates the problem of permeability pulmonary oedema ('ventilator lung/oxygen toxicity'). A variety of lung-protective ventilatory techniques have been developed to overcome these problems. **Permissive hypercapnia** is a technique which allows the patient to have a high $Paco_2$ level (e.g. 10 kPa; 75 mmHg) in order to reduce the alveolar ventilation and to avoid excessive airway pressure. **Inverse ratio ventilation** prolongs the inspiratory phase of ventilation such that it is longer than the expiratory phase allowing the tidal volume to be delivered over a longer time at a lower pressure. However, this may cause progressive air trapping. **High-frequency jet ventilation** is a technique whereby small volumes are delivered as an injected jet of gas at high frequencies (e.g. 100–300/min). Ventilation of the patient in the **prone posture** may be beneficial as it reduces gravity-dependent fluid deposition and atelectasis. **Extra corporeal membrane oxygenation** (ECMO) involves the diversion of the patient's circulation through an artificial external membrane to provide oxygen and remove carbon dioxide. None of these ventilatory strategies has yet achieved a major improvement in the overall prognosis of ARDS but each may be useful in individual circumstances.

Optimising haemodynamic function

Reducing the pulmonary artery pressure may help to reduce the degree of pulmonary capillary leak. This is achieved by avoiding excessive fluid administration, by judicious use of **diuretics** and by use of drugs which act as **vasodilators** of the pulmonary arteries. Treatment is sometimes guided by use of a balloon-tipped pulmonary artery catheter (Swan–Ganz) which measures pulmonary artery pressures, pulmonary capillary wedge pressure (reflecting left atrial pressure) and cardiac output (using a thermal dilution technique). Haemodynamic management essentially consists of achieving an **optimal balance** between a **low pulmonary artery pressure** to reduce fluid leak to the alveoli, an **adequate systemic blood pressure** to maintain perfusion of tissues and organs (e.g. kidneys) with a satisfactory **cardiac output** and optimal **oxygen delivery** to tissues (oxygen delivery is a function of the haemoglobin level, oxygen saturation of blood and cardiac output). Most drugs used to vasodilate the pulmonary arteries, such as nitrates or calcium antagonists, also cause systemic vasodilatation with hypotension and impaired organ perfusion. Inotropes and vasopressor agents, such as **dobutamine** or **norepinephrine** (noradrenaline) may be needed to maintain systemic blood pressure and cardiac output particularly in patients with the sepsis syndrome (caused by septicaemia or peritonitis, for example) in which sepsis is associated with systemic vasodilatation. Inhaled **nitric oxide** (NO) may be used as a selective pulmonary artery vasodilator. Because it is given by inhalation it is selectively distributed to ventilated regions of the lung where it produces vasodilatation. This vasodilatation to ventilated alveoli may significantly improve ventilation/perfusion matching with improved gas exchange. NO is rapidly inactivated by haemoglobin preventing a systemic action. It is necessary to monitor the level of inspired gas, nitrogen dioxide (NO_2) and methaemoglobin to avoid toxicity.

General management

Correction of anaemia by **blood transfusions** improves oxygen carriage in the blood and oxygen delivery to the tissues. **Nutritional support** (e.g. by enteral feeding via a jejunostomy) is crucial in maintaining the patient's overall fitness in the face of critical illness, and correction of hypoalbuminaemia improves the osmotic pressure of the plasma reducing fluid leak from the circulation. The ventilated patient with ARDS is particularly vulnerable to **nosocomial pneumonia** and bronchoalveolar lavage may be helpful in identifying pathogens. **Multiorgan failure** often complicates ARDS requiring further specific interventions (e.g. dialysis for renal failure).

Anti-inflammatory therapies

A key target for potential treatment is the cascade of inflammatory events arising from the tissue damage resulting from the initiating illness. Unfortunately, these events are poorly understood and no anti-inflammatory drug has yet achieved an established role in treating ARDS. Corticosteroids have not been beneficial. Ibuprofen has been used in an attempt to reduce neutrophil activation and pentoxifylline has been used because of its action in reducing the production of interleukin-1. Haemofiltration is a procedure primarily used to control fluid balance but it may have an additional beneficial effect in patients with sepsis by removal of endotoxins. Recently it has been recognised that there is a link between the coagulation system and the immune response to sepsis with activation of cytokines, neutrophils, monocytes, complement, coagulation and fibrinolytic systems as part of the systemic inflammatory response to infection. Recombinant human activated protein C has an anti-inflammatory effect by blocking the production of cytokines and cell adhesion and by inhibiting thrombin production. This drug has been shown to reduce mortality when used early in the treatment of patients with severe sepsis and multiple organ failure.

Prognosis

Despite intensive research into the inflammatory mechanisms giving rise to ARDS and major advances in ventilatory techniques and haemodynamic control, the mortality of patients with ARDS remains very high at >50%. Patients who survive may be left with lung fibrosis and impaired gas diffusion but some patients make a remarkably full recovery despite having been critically ill with gross lung injury requiring prolonged treatment in ITU.

Keypoints

- ARDS is a form of acute pulmonary oedema due to increased endothelial permeability caused by an inflammatory response to illness or injury.
- Precipitating factors include systemic sepsis, trauma, burns, pancreatitis and aspiration of gastric contents.
- Patients are severely hypoxic with diffuse infiltrates on chest X-ray with no evidence of cardiac failure.
- Treatment involves correction of the initiating illness and supportive care using lung-protective ventilation with PEEP.

Further reading

Artigas A. Epidemiology and prognosis of acute respiratory distress syndrome. *Eur Resp Mon* 2002; **20**: 1–21.

Ashbaugh DG, Bigelow DB, Petty TL, Levine BE. Acute respiratory distress in adults. *Lancet* 1967; **ii**: 319–23.

Baudouin S, Evans T. Improving outcomes for severely ill medical patients. *Clin Med* 2002; **2**: 92–4.

Bernard GR. Acute respiratory distress syndrome: a historical perspective. *Am J Resp Crit Care Med* 2005; **172**: 798–806.

Bernard GR, Artigas A, Brigham KL et al. Report of the American–European Consensus Conference on ARDS. *Intens Care Med* 1994; **20**: 225–32.

MacIntyre NR. Current issues in mechanical ventilation for respiratory failure. *Chest* 2005; **128** (Suppl.): 561–7.

Matthay MA, Zimmerman GA. Acute lung injury and acute respiratory distress syndrome. *Am J Resp Cell Mol Biol* 2005; **33**: 319–27.

Tighe D, Moss R, Bennett D. The history of trauma and its relationship to the adult respiratory distress syndrome. *Br J Intens Care* 1996; **6**: 272–4.

Vincent JL, Abraham E. The last 100 years of sepsis. *Am J Resp Crit Care Med* 2006; **173**: 256–63.

Chapter 19

Sleep-related breathing disorders

Introduction

People spend almost one-third of their lives asleep but it is only relatively recently that we have become aware of the important effects of sleep on respiratory physiology, and of specific breathing disorders occurring during sleep, such as the obstructive sleep apnoea syndrome (OSAS). The sleep disruption that results from OSAS has important consequences for the patient's quality of life in terms of daytime sleepiness, poor concentration and decreased cognitive function. It is now becoming clear that the diagnosis and treatment of OSAS also has major public health implications as OSAS is being increasingly recognised as a risk factor for cardiovascular disease, stroke and hypertension and a significant cause of accidents at home, at work and on the road.

Sleep physiology

Although familiar to everyone as a state in which the eyes are closed, postural muscles relaxed and consciousness suspended, sleep is an enigmatic condition which has essential refreshing and restorative effects on the mind and body. Electroencephalogram (EEG) studies show that sleep may be divided into five stages and two major categories. Stages 1–4 are characterised by loss of alpha wave activity and progressive slowing in the frequency with increase in the amplitude of the EEG wave form,

and during these stages rapid eye movements are absent: **non-REM sleep**. Stage 5 is characterised by rapid eye movement: **REM sleep**. Typically, a person drifts from an awake relaxed state into sleep, progressing serially through EEG stages 1–4, becoming less responsive to stimuli and less rousable. After about 70 minutes of non-REM sleep the person usually enters a period of deep sleep associated with rapid eye movements. This usually lasts about 30 minutes and is often followed by a brief awakening and a return to stage 1 sleep. Cycles of REM and non-REM sleep continue throughout the night with the period spent in REM sleep becoming longer, such that it occupies about 25% of total sleep time. During REM sleep the person is difficult to rouse and has reduced muscle tone. This stage of sleep is associated with dreaming and a variety of autonomic changes including penile erection and changes in respiration, blood pressure, pulse rate and pupil diameter. Irregularity of respiration and heart rate are common in this stage of sleep and apnoeic episodes lasting 15–20 seconds are common in normal individuals. The exact sleep 'architecture' (depth, character and changes) varies with age and circumstances (e.g. unfamiliar environment, disruption of regular routine), so that it can be difficult to define precisely normal and abnormal patterns by arbitrary cut-off points. Although sleep has major beneficial effects on the mind and body, the physiological changes during sleep may aggravate pre-existing

Chapter 20

Smoking and smoking cessation

Introduction

In the UK there are about 13 million smokers and half of these will die prematurely of disease caused by smoking, losing an average of 8 years of life. Cigarette smoking is the largest single preventable cause of death and disability in the UK. Smoking prevention and smoking cessation are among the most vital interventions which doctors, nurses and all health-care workers can achieve in improving the health of their patients.

History of smoking

Tobacco was introduced to Europe around 1500. Initially, most tobacco was sold for pipes, cigars, chewing and snuff. The commercial manufacture and promotion of cigarettes started around 1900 and cigarette smoking had become popular with men by the time of World War I and with women by World War II. **By the 1940s about 70% of men and 40% of women smoked** (Fig. 20.1). At that time smoking was very fashionable and its health

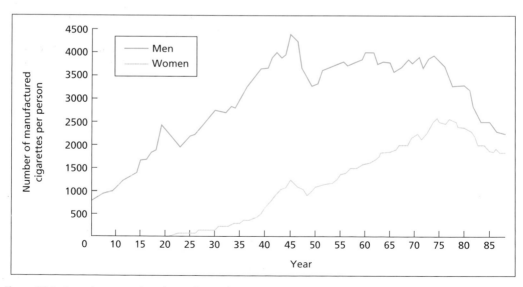

Figure 20.1 Annual consumption of manufactured cigarettes per person, UK, 1905–87. (Reproduced with permission from the Lung and Asthma Information Agency Factsheet 98/2.)

effects had not yet been recognised. In the 1950s an epidemic of lung cancer was becoming apparent and studies, such as those of Doll and Hill, established the causative link between cigarette smoking and lung cancer. In the early 1960s the Royal College of Physicians in London and the Surgeon General of the USA published landmark reports documenting the causal relationship between smoking and lung cancer. Cigarette smoking by men increased until the mid 1940s when it started to decrease, with a more rapid decline occurring from the 1970s onwards (Fig. 20.2). Smoking trends of women followed those of men about 25 years later. Peak consumption by women occurred in the 1970s, leading to the current epidemic of lung cancer in women in the UK and USA. **At present about 29% of men and 28% of women smoke** so that equality of the sexes has occurred. Individuals from the lower socioeconomic groups have higher rates of smoking and this is an important factor in the overall adverse effect of social class on mortality and morbidity.

Although the prevalence of smoking has been falling in developed countries, there has been a dramatic increase in smoking in the developing countries. **Globally** it is estimated that there are **1100 million smokers** (about 30% of the adult population). As stricter controls on tobacco were being enforced in the developed world over recent decades, cigarettes were being actively promoted in China, India and the African countries. It is now estimated, for example, that there are 300 million smokers in China where 61% of men smoke. The epidemic of smoking-related mortality and morbidity that has dominated health trends in the Western world in the last century is likely to be repeated on a massive scale in the developing world in the next 100 years.

Health effects of smoking

Worldwide about **4 million people die annually from tobacco-related illnesses** at present. By 2030 it is estimated that this will rise to 10 million deaths each year and that 70% of these deaths will be in the developing world. In the UK 50 000 deaths from **cancer** are attributed to smoking each year. Cancer of the lung, mouth, larynx, oesophagus, stomach,

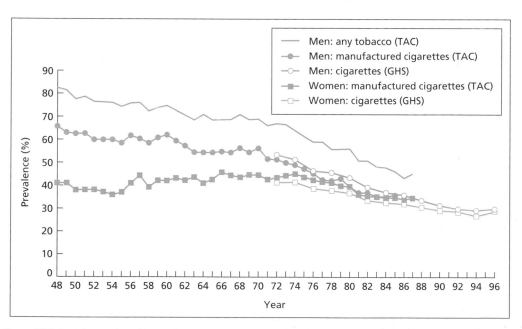

Figure 20.2 Prevalence of smoking in the UK, 1948–96. TAC, tobacco advisory council survey; GHS, general household survey. (Reproduced with permission from the Lung and Asthma Information Agency Factsheet 98/2.)

pancreas and kidney are all causally linked to smoking. Smokers have twice the risk of death from cancers of non-smokers (see Chapter 13). Smoking is the main cause of **chronic obstructive pulmonary disease** (COPD), with about 12 5000 new cases developing each year in the UK (see Chapter 12). Up to 50% of cases of **coronary heart disease** are attributed to smoking. Smoking increases the risk of **stroke** by up to threefold. About 90% of patients with **peripheral vascular disease** are smokers. Smoking during pregnancy doubles the risk of having a **low-birth weight baby** and increases the risk of complications such as premature labour, miscarriage and stillbirth.

Passive smoking

Breathing other people's tobacco smoke—passive smoking—has been shown to have a number of biological effects including increased blood leucocyte counts, release of oxidants by stimulated neutrophils and elevated urinary cotinine (a metabolite of nicotine) levels, so that there is no doubt that non-smokers can inhale significant amounts of smoke from the environment. Irritant effects (e.g. eye, nose, throat symptoms) constitute a nuisance to those exposed to environmental tobacco smoke so that smoking is often banned in public places such as restaurants, airplanes, buses and workplaces. In theory, passive smoking could cause any of the health effects associated with active smoking but at a level of risk significantly less than that of active smoking. Non-smokers who live with a smoker have the greatest exposure to the effects of environmental tobacco smoke. This is particularly the case for children whose parents smoke at home. For example, a woman who has never smoked has an estimated **24% greater risk of developing lung cancer and a 30% greater risk of developing ischaemic heart disease** if she lives with a smoker. Children who are exposed to environmental tobacco smoke at home have an increased risk of bronchitis, lower respiratory infections and exacerbations of asthma. Occupational exposure to tobacco smoke is a hazard to those working in ⁀laces such as bars, restaurants and nightclubs, and ⁀ng bans are being introduced in many places

as part of the requirement to provide a safe working environment.

Composition of smoke

Cigarette smoke has a very complex composition, with gas and particulate phase components. The smoke emitted from the burning end of the cigarette is known as **'sidestream' smoke** and emerges directly into the environment, whereas the **'mainstream' smoke** is inhaled directly by the smoker. Many toxic constituents are present in higher concentrations in sidestream smoke, and this may be important in assessing the risks of passive smoking. **Tar** consists of a mixture of aromatic hydrocarbons including carcinogens such as nitrosamines, aromatic amines and benzopyrene, and is the component linked to the development of lung cancer. **Carbon monoxide** is associated with the cardiovascular risks of smoking and **nicotine** has addictive properties. Both the gas and particulate components of cigarette smoke are implicated in the development of COPD. From the 1950s onward, when filtered cigarettes began to replace unfiltered varieties, the tar yield fell by about half and the nicotine yield fell by about one-third, but the carbon monoxide yield remained stable. However, changes in the contents of cigarettes cause many smokers to inhale more deeply or to smoke more cigarettes, and it is not possible to produce a 'safe' cigarette because smoking involves the burning of complex hydrocarbons that will always produce toxic products.

Smoking cessation

The process of smoking cessation may be divided into five stages:
- **Precontemplation** (contented smoker not considering cessation).
- **Contemplation** (concerned smoker who would like to stop).
- **Preparation** (smoker planning practical ways of stopping).
- **Action** (setting a quit date).
- **Maintenance** (supporting cessation and preventing relapse).

People who smoke need **help, not hostility** from health-care workers in stopping smoking and it is important to develop a therapeutic partnership which provides **support** and **practical advice**. Smoking is such an important health issue that all health-care workers should routinely ask patients about their smoking status and advise them appropriately—**'All the As'**.

- **Ask** about smoking at every opportunity and document the smoking status of all patients. **Applaud** those who are non-smokers. **Assess** the **attitude** of smokers to smoking cessation. Some say that they do not intend to quit and these should be advised to contemplate the health risk. Such **advice** should be individualised to their current health issues (e.g. asthma, respiratory infections) or social circumstances (e.g. plans to become pregnant). Young people often erroneously think that they will have time to stop smoking later if diseases develop. Sometimes 'shock tactics' may help them contemplate the future (e.g. when your daughter is getting married in 20 years' time who will walk her down the aisle if you get lung cancer?). About 70% of smokers say that they would like to quit and these need to be encouraged to move from contemplation of stopping to taking **action** to stop.
- **Advise** all smokers on the value of stopping, the risks to health of continuing and the support available in helping them to stop (e.g. nicotine replacement therapy). **Assure** them that 'It's never too late to stop' and encourage them to 'Never stop trying to stop'.
- **Assist** patients who have decided to stop with practical personalised advice and support. Set a **quit date** and stop completely on that day. Plan ahead by identifying problems and situations where the temptation to smoke arises (e.g. after meals, in the pub, during coffee breaks at work). Enlist the support of family and friends. Encourage them not to rely solely on 'will power' but to consider using **nicotine replacement therapy**. Adopt a positive **attitude**: 'I know you can do it, and we will help'. Provide a booklet giving advice and practical tips for smoking cessation.
- **Arrange** follow-up and support. Offer a follow-up visit with the doctor or nurse about 1 week after the quit date. Applaud success and warn about preventing relapse.

More **intensive smoking cessation support** can help smokers who are motivated to stop but who have repeatedly failed. Group sessions with other smokers provide additional support and encouragement, and can be used to develop coping skills, training in dealing with cravings and social support.

Pharmacotherapy (Table 20.1)

Small doses of nicotine produce predominantly stimulant effects such as arousal, whereas larger doses produce mainly depressant effects such as relaxation and relief of stress. **Nicotine withdrawal** can cause irritability, restlessness, anxiety, insomnia and a craving for cigarettes. Nicotine replacement therapy approximately doubles the success rates of attempts at smoking cessation and smokers should be encouraged to use it to avoid withdrawal symptoms. Typically, a heavy smoker is given **transdermal nicotine patches** 21 mg/day for 4 weeks, reducing to 14 mg/day for 2 weeks and then 7 mg/day for 2 weeks. Most withdrawal symptoms have resolved within that period of time. The patch is applied to the skin each morning and delivers a constant dose over 16–24 hours, but the onset of action is quite slow. Patients who experience marked cravings for cigarettes may benefit from using nicotine **chewing gum, lozenges, inhalator** or **nasal spray** which provide more rapid peak blood levels from absorption of the nicotine through the buccal or nasal mucosa. Nicotine replacement therapy is safe, but is not recommended in pregnancy. Addiction to nicotine replacement therapy can occur in a few patients

Table 20.1 Pharmacotherapy in smoking cessation.

Nicotine replacement therapy
Transdermal patch
Chewing gum
Lozenges
Inhalator
Nasal spray
Bupropion (amfebutamone)

who use it in the long term, but most patients can be weaned off treatment over a few weeks. **Bupropion (amfebutamone)** is a newer antidepressant drug which significantly improves the success of attempts at smoking cessation, although its mode of action is uncertain. It has some significant side-effects, most notably a 1 in 1000 risk of epileptic seizures such that it is contraindicated in patients with convulsive disorders, central nervous system disease, bulimia or anorexia nervosa, and in patients experiencing symptoms of withdrawal from alcohol or benzodiazepines.

Primary prevention

Many long-term smokers were introduced to the habit as teenagers when they were vulnerable to cigarette advertising and when smoking may have been seen as a symbol of 'forbidden' adult behaviour. Measures designed to discourage smoking among young people are particularly important in the primary prevention of smoking-related diseases. Most young people are fully aware of the causal relationship of smoking and disease but they feel healthy, young and 'immortal' and do not relate well to concepts of ageing and disease. Counteracting this normal rebellious youth culture is difficult, but involves the promotion of a **positive image of a healthy lifestyle** and emphasising the **unattractiveness of the smoker**, whose clothes, hands and breath reek of tobacco ('It's like kissing an ashtray'). In teenagers sporting activities are inversely related to smoking because **sports** seem to promote self-confidence, encourage a healthy lifestyle and reduce peer influences about smoking. Mass media intervention, with **advertisements** promoting the anti-smoking

message targeted at the young, also appear to be effective in preventing the uptake of smoking. Outright prohibition of smoking is not likely to be feasible or successful but the examples of parents, teachers, sports people and society in general are crucial.

Tackling the epidemic of smoking-related mortality and morbidity requires action by all levels of society. There is a crucial role for all health-care workers in providing leadership and example in creating a tobacco-free society.

Keypoints

- Smoking is the largest single preventable cause of death and disability in the UK.
- Advice on smoking prevention is one of the most important interventions which health-care workers can achieve.
- Ask, advise, assist all smokers about smoking cessation at every opportunity.
- Nicotine replacement therapy helps smokers to quit.

Further reading

Edwards R. The problem of tobacco smoking. *BMJ* 2004; **328**: 217–19.

Jamrozik K. Estimated deaths attributable to passive smoking among UK adults: database analysis. *BMJ* 2005; **300**: 812–15.

Lung and Asthma Information Agency. *Trends in Smoking*. Factsheet 98/2, http://www.laia.ac.uk

Raw M, McNeill A, West R. Smoking cessation guidelines for health professionals. *Thorax* 1998; **53** (Suppl. 5): 1–38.

Srivastava P, Currie GP, Britton J. Smoking cessation. *BMJ* 2006; **332**: 1324–6.

Chapter 21

Lung transplantation

Introduction

Lung transplantation is now an established treatment option for some patients with end-stage lung disease who have failed to respond to maximum medical treatment. However, lung transplantation is associated with a high mortality and a limited long-term prognosis, and the critical shortage of donor organs severely restricts the application of the procedure. The first heart transplantation was performed in 1967 in Groote Schuur hospital, South Africa, when a man in end-stage cardiac failure received the heart of a young woman killed in a road traffic accident. Initial attempts at lung transplantation were unsuccessful but surgical advances, better selection of suitable patients and the introduction of ciclosporin immunosuppression introduced a new era, with the first successful heart–lung transplantation performed in 1981 in Stanford, USA, for a patient with primary pulmonary hypertension.

Types of operation

Surgical techniques have been developed to transplant a single lung, both lungs or the heart and lungs. Approximately 1600 procedures are performed every year worldwide.

Heart–lung transplant

The recipient's diseased lungs and heart are removed through a median sternotomy and the donor lungs and heart are implanted as a block. If the recipient's heart is normal it may be donated to another patient (domino procedure).

Single-lung transplant

A diseased lung is removed through a thoracotomy incision, leaving the heart and contralateral lung intact. The donor lung is then implanted using a bronchial anastomosis. The residual native lung must be free of infection or it will be a source of sepsis in the post-operative period when the patient is immunosuppressed, so that this procedure is not suitable for patients with cystic fibrosis, for example. The donor's heart and other lung are available to transplant to other patients.

Bilateral-lung transplant

- *Double-lung transplant*: the diseased lungs are removed through a median sternotomy, leaving the heart intact. The donor lungs are implanted as a block using a tracheal anastomosis.
- *Bilateral sequential single-lung transplant*: a transverse bilateral thoracotomy is performed dividing the sternum horizontally. The diseased lungs are removed and two separated lungs are implanted with separate bronchial anastomoses.

Donor organs are most commonly procured from patients who are less than 55 years of age who have suffered a catastrophic spontaneous intracranial haemorrhage or a major head injury who have

by the occurrence of bronchiolitis obliterans syndrome.

Future prospects

The shortage of donor organs and the occurrence of obliterative bronchiolitis are the two main problems to be overcome in lung transplantation. The general public are encouraged to carry **donor cards** in order to raise the general awareness of organ donation issues. However, less than 20% of cadaveric donors have lungs suitable for donation because the lungs of a ventilated brain dead patient are very vulnerable to infection, aspiration and lung injury. Management aimed at **optimising donor lung function** prior to retrieval and better identification of the criteria that make a lung unsuitable for donation might increase the number of useable organs. **Xenotransplantation** (the use of animal organs for transplantation in humans) has been unsuccessful because of hyper-acute rejection, and there are concerns about the potential for the spread of animal viruses to humans. **Lobar transplantation from living donors** has been undertaken for patients with cystic fibrosis whereby two living relatives, who have compatible blood groups, each donate a lobe which is of adequate size to fill a hemithorax of the recipient. There are concerns, however, about the risks of this procedure to the donors. It is hoped that developments in **immunosuppressive therapies** will reduce the occurrence of oblitera-tive bronchiolitis. These include total lymphoid irradiation and drugs such as tacrolimus, sirolimus, mycophenolate mofetil and ciclosporin microemul-sion formulations.

Further reading

Belkin RA, Henig NR, Singer LG et al. Risk factors for death of patients with cystic fibrosis awaiting

> ### Keypoints
>
> - Lung transplantation is now an established option for some patients with end-stage lung disease.
> - There is a critical shortage of donor organs.
> - The transplanted lungs are very vulnerable to infection and rejection.
> - Bronchiolitis obliterans syndrome is a form of chronic rejection which limits long-term survival.
> - Survival rates post-lung transplantation are 75% at 1 year and 55% at 5 years.

lung transplantation. *Am J Respir Crit Care Med* 2006; **173**: 659–66.

DePerrot M, Weder W, Patterson GA, Keshavjee S. Strategies to increase limited donor resources. *Eur Respir J* 2004; **23**: 477–82.

Duncan MD, Wilkes D. Transplant-related immunosuppression: a review of immunosuppression and pulmonary infections. *Proc Am Thoracic Soc* 2005; **2**: 449–55.

Estenne M, Kotloff RM. Update in transplantation 2005. *Am J Respir Crit Care Med* 2006; **173**: 593–8.

Kotloff RM, Ahya VN. Medical complications of lung transplantation. *Eur Respir J* 2004; **23**: 334–42.

Trulock EP, Edwards LB, Taylor DO et al. Registry of the international society of heart and lung transplantation report. *J Heart Lung Transplant* 2005; **24**: 956–7.

Yates B, Murphy DM, Forrest IA et al. Azithromycin reverses airflow obstruction in established bronchiolitis obliterans syndrome. *Am J Respir Crit Care Med* 2005; **172**: 772–5.

Index

Note: page numbers in *italics* refer to figures and those in **bold** refer to tables.